MedStudy®

Internal Medicine Board-Style Questions & Answers

2014

ANSWERS

Robert A. Hannaman, MD
Editor in Chief

TABLE OF CONTENTS

Disclaimers

IMPORTANT: These Q&A books are meant to be used as an adjunct to the MedStudy Internal Medicine Review Core Curriculum. The ABIM exams cover a vast realm of diagnostic and treatment knowledge. Board-simulation exercise such as these self-testing Q&As are valuable tools, but these alone are not adequate preparation for a Board exam. Be sure you use a comprehensive IM review resource such as the MedStudy Core Curriculum in addition to these Q&As for adequate exam preparation.

Content: The primary purpose of this activity is educational. Medicine and accepted standards of care are constantly changing. We at MedStudy do our best to review and include in this activity accurate discussions of the standards of care, methods of diagnosis, and selection of treatments. However, the authors/presenters, editors, advisors, and publisher—and all other parties involved with the preparation of this work—disclaim any guarantee that the information contained in this activity and its associated materials is in every respect accurate or complete. MedStudy further disclaims any and all liability for damages and claims that may result from the use of information or viewpoints presented. We recommend you confirm the information contained in this activity and in any other educational material with current sources of medical knowledge whenever considering actual clinical presentations or treating patients.

ABIM: For over 20 years, MedStudy has excelled in determining and teaching what a clinically competent Internal Medicine physician should know. The American Board of Internal Medicine (ABIM) tests this exact same pool of knowledge. MedStudy's expertise, demonstrated by the superb pass rate of those who use it in their studies, is in the actual "teaching" of this knowledge in a clear, learner-friendly manner that results in a stronger knowledge base, improved clinical skills, and better Board results. Although what we teach is in sync with what the Boards test, MedStudy has no affiliation with the ABIM, and our authors, editors, and reviewers have no access to ABIM exam content. Our material is developed as original work by MedStudy physician authors, with additional input from expert contributors, based on their extensive backgrounds in professional medical education. This content is designed to include subject matter typically tested in certification and recertification exams as outlined in the ABIM's publicly available exam blueprints but makes no use of, and divulges no details of, ABIM's proprietary exam content.

A note on editorial style: MedStudy uses a standardized approach to the naming of diseases. The previous method of naming was to use the possessive form that adds "'s" to the names of diseases and disorders, such as Lou Gehrig's disease, Klinefelter's syndrome, and others. In MedStudy material, you will see the non-possessive form when the proper name is followed by a common noun; e.g., "This patient would warrant workup for Crohn disease." Exceptions to the possessive form include Bell's palsy and Still's murmur. The possessive form will be used, however, when an entity is referred to solely by its proper name without a following common noun; e.g., "The symptoms are classic for Crohn's." The *AMA Manual of Style*, *JAMA*®, and *Scientific Style and Format* are among the publications that promote and use the non-possessive form for all disease names.

MEDSTUDY
1455 Quail Lake Loop
Colorado Springs, CO 80906
(800) 841-0547
www.medstudy.com

About the questions and answers in this learning activity

The questions, answers, and explanations in this learning activity are developed by specialty and subspecialty experts who are additionally physician educators.

The questions in this book are reflective of the questions on the Board exams. As a result, you will find that the percentage of questions by topic in this activity mirrors the Board template. You will find questions of varying length here. The very short ones are designed to nail home an important point you need to know and remember for your Boards. The lengthier questions help you integrate content on a subject with additional clinical information to better simulate a real-life patient scenario. This helps you recognize disease states and associated treatment, which is a skill heavily tested on Board exams. Some selected patient case scenarios may appear more than once with only slight variations, with the associated questions addressing different diagnoses and treatment aspects of the case. This is in keeping with the approach Board questions take in limiting patient case assessments to one key testing point.

In short, this Q&A material is designed to impart not only relevant knowledge for IM Board exams but also challenge your skills in interpretation and intervention, which is what Board exams attempt to assess. This is why we call these, appropriately, "Board-style" questions and answers.

There is a popular misconception that members of organizations perceived to be associated with medical boards write Board exam questions; e.g., ACP/MKSAP with the American Board of Internal Medicine or AAP/PREP with the American Board of Pediatrics. Not only is this not true, it is actually forbidden for anyone to write formal Board exam questions if they work for a company or organization in the business of producing Board preparation materials. This would compromise the integrity of the examining process.

MedStudy is proud to be able to bring you Board-style questions and answers of the highest quality—to offer you education that is relevant in a format that reinforces your knowledge to prepare you well for whatever challenge the ABIM Board exam presents to you. One final note: Even the best question-and-answer exercise by itself is not an adequate preparation for a Board exam. These Q&As should be used as an adjunct to a comprehensive Board review course—such as MedStudy's Internal Medicine Review Core Curriculum. The Boards cover a vast realm of information that Board simulation Q&As alone cannot encompass.

GASTROENTEROLOGY

1. Answer: C

Answer: Perform endoscopy.

This patient presents with symptoms characteristic of GERD for the last 3 months. In performing an evaluation on patients with GERD symptoms, it is important to recognize "alarm symptoms," which include dysphagia, anemia, weight loss, and vomiting. This patient has anemia noted on his laboratory studies. The next best step would be upper endoscopy. Had alarm symptoms been absent, an empiric trial with a PPI would be appropriate. An ambulatory pH study would be indicated in patients with GERD who do not respond to empiric therapy. Testing for *H. pylori* would be indicated in patients with dyspepsia (burning, epigastric pain, bothersome postprandial fullness, early satiety). Tissue transglutaminase IgA Ab would be indicated to evaluate for celiac disease. Manifestations of celiac disease can include abdominal pain and anemia. However, celiac disease should present with signs of malabsorption, which this patient does not have.

Board Testing Point: Recognize alarm symptoms that warrant endoscopic evaluation in patients with GERD.

2. Answer: A

Answer: EGD.

This patient likely has uncomplicated reflux disease, but her family history of GI cancer, blood in her stool, and dysphagia are all "alarm" symptoms that merit workup. The patient needs more than just medication or reassurance at this point, though the workup is still likely to be negative. EGD is the correct answer. Barium esophagram could be considered, but her dysphagia only to solids is concerning for a stricture, and limiting her diagnostic/therapeutic evaluation to EGD with possible dilation would probably be the best course of action.

Board Testing Point: Recognize the alarm signals in GERD.

3. Answer: D

Answer: Serum lipase.

The patient in this question has acute pancreatitis, manifested by abdominal pain with associated nausea/vomiting. His physical exam reveals Cullen sign, ecchymotic bruising in the periumbilical region that is an uncommon finding associated with pancreatitis. However, this is not a diagnostic finding. The next best step would be to confirm the diagnosis of acute pancreatitis by an elevated serum lipase or amylase level. A CT of the abdomen should be reserved for cases where the diagnosis remains unclear after initial lab work. An ultrasound of the abdominal aorta would be used if you suspected an abdominal aneurysm. ERCP would be indicated to treat a patient with confirmed gallstone pancreatitis. CA 19-9 is a nonspecific serum test used in the diagnosis of cholangiocarcinoma and has no role in the diagnosis of acute pancreatitis.

Board Testing Point: Identify the clinical and laboratory features to diagnose acute pancreatitis.

4. Answer: E

Answer: Alcohol.
The patient in this question has acute pancreatitis, manifested by abdominal pain with associated nausea/vomiting and elevated lipase level. Gallstones are the most common precipitant of acute pancreatitis, but this patient has a history of remote cholecystectomy that makes this answer unlikely. After gallstones, alcohol is the next most common cause, accounting for up to 30% of cases in the United States. Tobacco is more commonly associated with chronic pancreatitis rather than acute pancreatitis. Hydrochlorothiazide has been linked with elevations in serum calcium and pancreatitis, but the incidence is much more uncommon compared to alcohol and gallstone pancreatitis. Hypertriglyceridemia is an infrequent cause of acute pancreatitis, accounting for approximately 1–3% of episodes.

Board Testing Point: Recall the most common etiologies of acute pancreatitis.

5. Answer: C

Answer: He had a recent MI.
Note that he should receive an EGD, except that his recent MI is a contraindication. His use of ASA is not a contraindication nor is his platelet count. Other contraindications for an EGD include an uncooperative or combative patient or an intestinal perforation (which requires immediate surgical intervention, not an EGD).

Board Testing Point: Know the contraindications for EGD.

6. Answer: A

Answer: Endoscopic retrograde cholangiopancreatography (ERCP) with laparoscopic cholecystectomy.
Complications of gallstones include acute cholecystitis, biliary colic, gallstone ileus, fistula formation, porcelain gallbladder caused by calcium and salt deposition in the wall, and stones in the common bile duct, which occur in up to 10–15% of patients. Occult duct stones remaining after cholecystectomies can occur in up to 1–5% of patients. Rarely, primary stones will occur in the ducts in the setting of increased pigment or congenital abnormalities.

This patient has symptoms of acute cholangitis (Charcot triad: biliary colic, jaundice, and fever with chills). Cholangitis is inflammation of the bile ducts usually caused by bacteria and most often occurs when there are gallstones partially obstructing the bile tract. Many patients with this condition respond rapidly with appropriate supportive measures, including antibiotics. The concern is when a complete obstruction of the ductal system occurs, which can lead to severe illness with resulting SIRS (systemic inflammatory response syndrome) or septic shock.

The most appropriate diagnostic study for choledocholithiasis (gallstones) is cholangiography, which usually is accomplished by ERCP with combined laparoscopic cholecystectomy. This reduces the risk of complicated biliary tract disease with the need for choledocholithotomy and T-tube drainage.

Ultrasound and MRCP would not be appropriate for an urgent scenario. Liver Bx would not be appropriate.

One other pearl from this case: A palpable gallbladder (Courvoisier sign) would suggest carcinoma of the pancreas.

Board Testing Point: Know that ERCP with laparoscopic cholecystectomy is the best therapeutic procedure for choledocholithiasis.

7. Answer: A

Answer: Esophagogastroduodenoscopy (EGD).
She has warning signs: new-onset dysphagia with weight loss in a smoker. In younger people with gradual onset, most would do barium swallow first. However, this woman is older and has abrupt-onset dysphagia with weight loss. MRI of chest is not indicated at this point. The Tensilon® test would be considered if you thought she had myasthenia gravis, but she has no symptoms of this besides dysphagia. Motility studies would be considered if the EGD is unremarkable; or more likely a CT scan of the chest would be the next step after the EGD shows her mass lesion.

Board Testing Point: Recognize the clinical warning signs when EGD would be the best test to work up dysphagia.

8. Answer: D

Answer: Achalasia.
Achalasia may present at any age but usually occurs between the ages of 50 and 60. Regurgitation while bending is common. Usually the regurgitation is **not** associated with heartburn, as is seen with gastroesophageal reflux. Chest pain can occur and in some patients can be severe. Treatment is focused at opening the lower esophageal sphincter. Initially, this can be done with pneumatic dilatation with a large balloon inserted within the LES. Surgical intervention via myotomy is also effective. Botulinum toxin has been used, but has a higher relapse rate. The barium swallow here was quite helpful in that you can see a large dilated esophagus tapering to a beak-like narrowing at the lower end—the classic finding for achalasia.

Chagas disease could present this way, but you would need something in the travel history to help you. The "not to South America" clue should have keyed you in to discard this diagnosis. Gastroesophageal reflux could give you these symptoms, but the barium swallow is classic for achalasia, and would not be seen with reflux disease. The CXR is also helpful since this is a classic description for this disease too. Esophageal ulcers more commonly present with retrosternal chest pain, odynophagia, or epigastric pain. Acute bleeding could be the only symptom. Again, in this patient, ulcer is not likely based on the clinical and x-ray findings. Finally, the Plummer-Vinson syndrome is when you see formation of an **anterior** web at the upper end of the esophagus; the x-ray findings do not support this syndrome.

Board Testing Point: Recognize the clinical and radiologic features of achalasia.

9. Answer: C

Answer: Progression is likely to occur, and stricture formation with nearly complete loss of peristalsis will be seen in later forms of this disease.
This woman has scleroderma. Over 80% of patients have involvement of the esophagus. It causes reduced-to-absent lower esophageal sphincter pressure (unlike achalasia). The other symptoms and signs that she has go along with the disease. The symptoms will not improve as the disease progresses. H2 blockers may provide some symptom relief but are unlikely to provide complete recovery from this progressive connective tissue disease. Her skin findings are related to her esophageal disease. The gastrointestinal findings frequently involve other areas besides the esophagus.

Board Testing Point: Recognize the clinical features of scleroderma and the associated gastroenterological manifestations.

10. Answer: D

Answer: Pill-induced esophagitis.
In adolescents, pill-induced esophagitis is common, especially if they do not take the time to use water to swallow pills. Doxycycline is one of the classic drugs to do this. Other common drugs associated with this include aspirin, NSAIDs such as ibuprofen, iron pills, potassium supplements, and alendronate (for post-menopausal osteoporosis). Scleroderma is very unlikely in a 16-year-old male without other symptoms. Gastroesophageal reflux would not generally cause this type of isolated symptom. Cocaine abuse is not associated with isolated dysphagia. Bulimia could be associated with dysphagia, but he has no other signs or symptoms of this illness.

Board Testing Point: Recognize the clinical characteristics of pill-induced esophagitis.

11. Answer: E

Answer: Improvement with therapeutic trial of anti-GERD medication.
All of the findings listed except improvement with therapy should prod you to get an EGD fairly quickly. They are the "alarm signals." Particularly worrisome in this patient is the heme-positive stool on rectal exam. The patient's alcohol and tobacco use also increases her likelihood of having gastrointestinal disease.

Board Testing Point: Know the "alarm signals" that warrant EGD.

12. Answer: B

Answer: He has severe disease that will likely require long-term medical therapy, so the best option is chronic proton pump inhibitor therapy.
The 2008 GERD guidelines recommend medical therapy over surgical intervention because of the inherent risks of surgery and the potential for increased side effects such as bloating and GI discomfort after surgery. It is unlikely that his GERD, severe as it is, will improve or "resolve over time." Because of its side effects (tachyphylaxis, lethargy, extrapyramidal effects, etc.), metoclopramide **cannot** be used long-term. As he has already shown, non-proton pump inhibitors are not likely to be effective. Omeprazole or another proton pump inhibitor could be used for long-term therapy and is an option.

Board Testing Point: Know that the latest GERD guidelines recommend medical therapy over surgical intervention because of the inherent risks of surgery and the potential for increased side effects.

13. Answer: D

Answer: Refer for surgery.
Now that he has high-grade dysplasia, he has 2 options according to the latest guidelines on Barrett esophagus published in 2008. The first option is standard resectional surgery, and the second option is to repeat EGD within 3 months and then follow 3-month EGD surveillance until intervention is needed. At this stage, decreasing gastric acid concentrations will not reverse the current damage; also, a 1-month time interval will not be useful in looking for changes. Surveillance every 6 months is too long a period of time in between. Monthly EGD is not cost-effective and very impractical. Finally, application of low-grade beam radiation to the affected area is not indicated and would harm the patient.

Board Testing Point: Know the latest guidelines for management of Barrett esophagus.

14. Answer: A

Answer: Since she has known *Helicobacter pylori,* it is prudent to treat her with appropriate antimicrobial therapy.
This is a difficult problem. In the first place, she never should have taken the test. The problem is what to do with this information. We know that *H. pylori* colonizes in most people without causing any disease. Therefore, you would think that further investigation is not indicated or necessary because she is asymptomatic, so no treatment is required. However, *H. pylori* is classified by the World Health Organization International Agency for Research on Cancer as a **definite** carcinogen.

Here is the problem: Even though it is very unlikely she will ever develop complications from her *H. pylori,* she should receive appropriate therapy. The testing done today is usually quite specific and sensitive for the infection, so wasting money on a new test is not likely to be helpful. She is completely asymptomatic, and we know that most people with *H. pylori* are asymptomatic, so any type of testing such as barium swallow or endoscopy is not indicated.

Board Testing Point: Know that finding *H. pylori* should result in initiation of therapy.

15. Answer: A

Answer: Non-invasive testing for *Helicobacter pylori.*
In a healthy young person (defined by the American Society of Gastroenterology as being anyone under the age of 45—complain to them if you are over 45!) with no "alarm" symptoms/signs, non-invasive *Helicobacter pylori* testing (without EGD) is indicated because the risk of gastric carcinoma is low. Indications for early EGD are anorexia, dysphagia, gastrointestinal bleeding (gross or occult), new-onset symptoms in persons > 45 years old, presence of a mass, unexplained anemia, unexplained weight loss, or severe vomiting. Non-invasive testing in symptomatic patients and treatment in those with positive results are cost-effective. Remember: Barium swallow is a test for dysphagia, **not** dyspepsia. EGD with biopsy **is** the most specific test for diagnosis of *H. pylori*-induced peptic ulcer disease, but is rarely indicated as the initial diagnostic test in uncomplicated ulcer disease in a young healthy person. On the biopsy specimen, you can actually look for histological evidence of the little critter (*H. pylori*) or do the rapid urease test on the specimen. Both are very specific for infection if present.

Remember that if this were an older person (> 45 years), you would proceed to EGD with biopsy of suspicious lesions. So remember: under 45 ... no EGD; over 45 … EGD for peptic ulcer workup. Finally, empirical H-2 blocker therapy alone would be ineffective for *H. pylori* infection.

Board Testing Point: Know the indications for non-invasive *H. pylori* testing.

16. Answer: D

Answer: A urea breath test is indicated at this point to determine cure.
About 75% of patients presumed to have uncomplicated peptic ulcer disease due to *H. pylori* infection are cured after 1 course of therapy. Treatment failure in the remainder of patients usually means that the ulcer will recur. Also, if untreated, these patients are at increased risk of complication such as gastrointestinal hemorrhage. The urea breath test is the best test to assess cure. A stool antigen test can also be used if the urea breath test is unavailable.

Repeating EGD is indicated only in certain instances: 1) persistent symptoms after 1–2 courses of therapy; 2) patients with gastric ulcers; or 3) suspicion of gastric cancer.

Cure confirmation can be done at 4–6 weeks after completing therapy. Patients cannot be on proton pump inhibitors during breath urea testing because it interferes with the testing.

Serologic testing is not effective for follow-up testing and also is no longer recommended for initial diagnosis.

Board Testing Point: Recognize that a urea breath test (or other noninvasive test) is the best test to follow up and determine cure of *H. pylori* infection.

17. Answer: D

Answer: Fasting serum gastrin level.
Several issues should make you think about Zollinger-Ellison syndrome (ZES). Note that his ulcer is in an unusual location; generally, any ulcer past the duodenal bulb should make you think about ZES. Also, he has severe esophagitis, which can be seen in regular ulcers; but the finding of the EGD makes ZES more likely. Additionally, his family history is quite strong, and he has been having diarrhea—another hallmark of this syndrome. Although diarrhea often occurs concomitantly with acid peptic disease, it may also occur **independent** of an ulcer. Etiology of the diarrhea is multifactorial, resulting from marked volume overload to the small bowel, pancreatic enzyme inactivation by acid, and damage to the intestinal epithelial surface by acid. Occasionally, you can have mild malabsorption of nutrients and vitamins. The diarrhea may also have a secretory component due to the direct stimulatory effect of gastrin on enterocytes or the co-secretion of additional hormones from the tumor, such as vasoactive intestinal peptide.

Gastric acid hypersecretion is responsible for the signs and symptoms observed in patients with ZES. Peptic ulcer is the most common clinical manifestation, occurring in over 90% of gastrinoma patients. Other clinical situations that should create suspicion of gastrinoma are ulcers refractory to standard medical therapy, ulcer recurrence after acid-reducing surgery, or ulcers presenting with frank complications (bleeding, obstruction, and perforation).

Board Testing Point: Recognize the clinical features of Zollinger-Ellison syndrome and know that a serum gastrin level is the best screening tool.

18. Answer: D

Answer: Alcohol consumption.
Note that alcohol consumption is **not** a risk factor for gastric carcinoma. All of the other factors listed are associated with increased risk. Also remember that history of gastric ulcer is **not** associated with increased risk of carcinoma. Other factors that are associated include diets high in dried, smoked, and salted foods; foods rich in nitrates; Barrett esophagus; and distal gastrectomy. Uranium mining is yet another association…so if they describe someone who is a uranium miner, look for the possibility of gastric carcinoma. Finally, lower socioeconomic class is associated with increased risk.

Board Testing Point: Know the risk factors for gastric carcinoma.

19. Answer: E

Answer: Colonoscopy with upper endoscopy.
She has symptoms consistent with Crohn disease. A colonoscopy with upper endoscopy will confirm disease location and show evidence of intestinal complications. Early in the disease process, the scope will show thickened folds and aphthous ulcerations. Later, "cobblestoning" occurs from longitudinal and transverse ulcerations, most frequently involving the small bowel. As the disease progresses, strictures and fistulas are

seen. Skip lesions are seen in Crohn disease. With her prolonged history and initial negative stool testing, it is not necessary to repeat ova and parasite testing again. An MRI would be helpful if you were concerned about an abscess; but her current symptoms are fairly mild, and no evidence exists for this. Endoscopic laparotomy is invasive and not indicated at this stage of diagnosis. A rectal biopsy is contraindicated and will not provide any helpful information for Crohn disease.

Board Testing Point: Recognize the clinical features of Crohn disease and know how to correctly evaluate and diagnose a patient with symptoms suggestive of Crohn's.

---

20. Answer: C

Answer: Stop sulfasalazine and use another agent for control of his disease.
Sulfasalazine is split into sulfapyridine and mesalamine. The problem is the sulfapyridine can cause reversible infertility in men. The best answer is to stop the sulfasalazine and prescribe another agent or attempt a trial off of therapy, since he has not had a problem in over 5 years. Once he has achieved "success," you could restart the sulfasalazine. Formal urologic evaluation is not indicated at this point; we have found that his sperm count is abnormally low, which explains why they are not conceiving. His wife does not need to undergo any testing. Also, since we have a reversible cause for his infertility and he is "functioning" properly, it is unnecessary to proceed with further workup, including testosterone levels. It wouldn't hurt to try boxers instead of briefs, but it is unlikely to make a difference in this case while his sperm count returns to normal.

Board Testing Point: Recognize that sulfasalazine may cause reversible infertility in men.

---

21. Answer: D

Answer: Recommend referral to surgery.
Even though he has been doing well until recently, the finding of high-grade dysplasia in flat mucosa indicates that colon cancer is possibly imminent, and removal of his complete colon will be curative. It is difficult to think about this in someone who has had relatively mild ulcerative colitis. Additionally, if you had found a mass lesion that showed dysplasia, complete colectomy would be indicated. Once you are at this stage, repeat colonoscopy is not helpful and will just prolong the inevitable. Likewise, reinstituting medical therapy would run the risk of allowing the high-grade dysplasia to progress.

Board Testing Point: Know the recommended colonic follow-up and treatment for patients with ulcerative colitis.

---

22. Answer: E

Answer: No antibiotic therapy.
With uncomplicated *Salmonella* gastroenteritis, antibiotic therapy is not indicated. If you treated her with antibiotics, you risk prolonging her shedding as well as increasing risk of resistance. Remember: *Shigella* you treat; *Salmonella* you generally don't. Exceptions are the very old, the very young, and the immunocompromised. We treat these special groups with antibiotics because the risk that the *Salmonella* may disseminate or cause more extensive problems is greater than the risk of prolonged shedding.

Board Testing Point: Know that *Salmonella* gastroenteritis generally does not require antibiotic therapy.

---

23. Answer: E

Answer: Give supportive care only.
Starting antibiotics in patients with *E. coli* O157:H7 actually **increases** the risk of HUS (hemolytic uremic syndrome). Therefore, supportive care is all that is indicated for this patient. Antibiotics are absolutely contraindicated!

Board Testing Point: Know that infection with *E. coli* O157:H7 is not treated with antibiotics.

24. Answer: A

Answer: *Campylobacter jejuni.*
This patient has classic Guillain-Barré syndrome, described as a syndrome that is idiopathic. However, *Campylobacter* enteritis is linked to about 1/3 of cases. The other organisms listed in the choices are not associated with this syndrome. Of note: As in this case, humans can get *Campylobacter* from their pets, especially dogs; conversely, dogs have become infected from their owners.

Board Testing Point: Recognize that *Campylobacter jejuni* is the most commonly associated diarrheal disease with development of Guillain-Barré syndrome.

25. Answer: C

Answer: Phenolphthalein abuse.
Note that she has a normal physical examination, and we have spent quite a bit of time and money on diagnostic tests, which all have been negative. The only positive laboratory value is the sodium hydroxide test, which indicates that she is abusing phenolphthalein. You can also confirm this with specific urine tests for this agent. The bisacodyl could be confirmed also by urine testing. Irritable bowel syndrome is a diagnosis of exclusion, and we have found another etiology for her symptoms. Carcinoid is a rare cause of diarrhea, but she does not have any of the other symptoms such as flushing, tachycardia, and explosive diarrhea. Colonoscopy and EGD are reserved for the later stage of workup of chronic diarrhea and are not indicated at this point, particularly in light of our findings of phenolphthalein abuse.

Board Testing Point: Recognize the clinical findings associated with phenolphthalein abuse.

26. Answer: D

Answer: Iron deficiency anemia.
Remember that iron is almost completely absorbed in the duodenum. With celiac disease, this is one of the main sites of malabsorption. B_{12} deficiency is very common with tropical sprue, but not celiac sprue. Folate deficiency is also common but less so than iron deficiency. Celiac disease exacerbation would not be responsible for anemia of this degree with heme-negative stools and no history of blood in the stool. Primary intestinal lymphoma is a rare late complication of celiac sprue—and the key words here are **rare** and **late**—so this is not a concern for this 40-year-old leprechaun at this point.

Board Testing Point: Recognize the association of iron deficiency anemia with celiac disease.

27. Answer: C

Answer: Infection with *Tropheryma whippeli.*
This patient has Whipple disease. Approximately 50% of the patients with Whipple's have generalized hyperpigmentation in association with diarrhea, weight loss, arthritis, and lymphadenopathy. Posterior uveitis is also seen. His night blindness is due to vitamin A deficiency from malabsorption—hence, the low carotene levels. The clincher was the biopsy of the small intestine and the findings in the lamina propria. Also available from certain labs is a PCR for the organism, which could be used on the biopsy material as well.

Board Testing Point: Know the clinical manifestations and the organism responsible for Whipple disease.

28. Answer: C

Answer: Colonoscopy every 5 years beginning now.
A positive family history is the most commonly identified factor that increases the risk of colorectal cancer. This gets a little confusing, so I will break it down in short paragraphs for you to "digest" more easily.

1. Persons with a single 1st degree relative with colorectal cancer that was diagnosed after age 60 experience a risk of colorectal cancer at age 40 that is equivalent to that of average-risk persons at age 50. Such persons should begin colorectal screening at age 40 (options for this: 1) colonoscopy every 10 years, or 2) annual fecal occult blood test plus flexible sigmoidoscopy every 5 years).

2. People at particularly increased risk are those with 2 or more 1st degree relatives with colorectal cancer or a single 1st degree relative diagnosed with colorectal cancer under the age of 60 (like this patient's father). The relatives of these affected patients should begin screening at age 40, or 10 years younger than the youngest affected 1st degree relative, whichever comes first. So, based on her family history and her dad's diagnosis at age 48, she should have started screening at age 38. Screening for these patients should be by colonoscopy at 3–5 year intervals depending on the strength of the family history.

Board Testing Point: Know the colorectal screening guidelines for individuals with a family history of colon cancer.

29. Answer: E

Answer: Repeat colonoscopy in 10 years.
Patients with hyperplastic polyps found on a screening colonoscopy require **no** further workup. These are quite common and do **not** predict increased prevalence of adenomas. CEA level is not indicated at all and is not approved as a screening test.

Board Testing Point: Recognize that small, hyperplastic polyps confer no increased risk of colon cancer.

30. Answer: D

Answer: Repeat colonoscopy in 3–6 months to be sure that resection was complete.
Large sessile polyps (> 2 cm) usually contain (as his did) villous tissue with a high malignant potential and tend to recur locally after resection. Frequently, these lesions cannot be completely or safely excised during colonoscopy, and the patient should be referred for primary surgical resection. However, in this case, complete excision was possible or thought possible, and it was done at time of colonoscopy. If a patient has had a successful colonoscopic excision of a large sessile polyp, then he/she should undergo follow-up colonoscopy 3–6 months later to determine whether the resection was complete. If a residual polyp is present at this point, it should be removed and the completeness of resection documented again within 3–6 months. If 2 or 3 attempts at removing a polyp are not successful, surgical referral is indicated.

Board Testing Point: Know the guidelines for follow-up of a suspicious sessile polyp.

31. Answer: E

Answer: Because the incidence of recurrent cancer is small, no other laboratory or imaging studies are indicated for this patient; follow-up should proceed as with benign adenomas.
He meets all of the favorable prognostic criteria outlined by the American College of Gastroenterology:

1) The polyp was completely excised and submitted *in toto* for evaluation.
2) The pathology lab fixed and sectioned the material to accurately determine the depth of invasion, grade of differentiation, and completeness of excision.
3) The cancer is not poorly differentiated.
4) There is no vascular or lymphatic involvement.
5) The margin of excision is not involved.

These patients with favorable prognostic criteria should have follow-up colonoscopy in 3 months to check for residual abnormal tissue at the polypectomy site if the polyp is sessile. After 1 negative examination, care can revert to standard surveillance as performed for patients with benign adenomas. Because the incidence of recurrent cancer is small, no other follow-up laboratory or imaging studies are indicated.

Board Testing Point: Know the guidelines for follow-up colonoscopy after finding a cancerous polyp.

32. Answer: D

Answer: Start adjuvant chemotherapy without radiation therapy.
She has Dukes C colon carcinoma or Stage III disease under newer staging methods (having 1–3 positive regional nodes places her in Stage III). The spread to the regional lymph nodes is what puts her in that category. Remember that Dukes A (Stage I) is cancer confined only to the mucosa and submucosa and requires surgical removal; Dukes B (Stage II) is cancer confined to the muscularis (B1) or through the serosa (B2), and generally requires surgical intervention only, although some would offer adjuvant 5-FU chemotherapy based on risk factors determined to be high-risk (poorly differentiated histology, lymphovascular/neural invasion, T4 lesion, perforation/obstruction, or fewer than 13 nodes obtained in the surgical specimen.) Dukes D (Stage IV) is with distant metastases and requires surgical intervention and expert guidance on whether adjuvant chemotherapy is helpful or not.

Board Testing Point: Know the recommended therapy for colon cancer based on the staging of the colon cancer.

33. Answer: B

Answer: Appendicitis.
Right lower quadrant pain with fever should always raise the suspicion for appendicitis. The typical presentation of appendicitis is initial peri-umbilical pain, which then localizes to the right lower quadrant. Fever and leukocytosis are also typical of appendicitis. The presentation of appendicitis in the elderly is often atypical. Pain can be poorly localized or even be absent. Fever may not be present. Leucocytosis is variable. Of patients older than 75 years of age, 80% present with atypical symptoms, as compared with 80% of patients younger than 65 years who present with typical symptoms. The rate of perforation is high in the elderly because of the delay in making a definite diagnosis of appendicitis. Appendicitis is still largely a clinical diagnosis. Computed tomography with colonic contrast has been reported to be 98% sensitive and 98% specific in experienced hands in diagnosing appendicitis. However, the sensitivity is variable depending on the radiologist, with sensitivity as low as 50%. The addition of intravenous contrast has been reported to increase sensitivity by about 25%.

Crohn disease is least likely for several reasons. Crohn disease is more prevalent in Caucasians than in African-Americans or Asians. It typically presents at an earlier age, with peak incidence at 15 to 35 years of age. The presentation is usually subacute with recurrent episodes of right lower quadrant abdominal pain, low-grade fever, diarrhea, and possibly a right lower quadrant mass. Acute ileitis, however, may have an abrupt onset with fever, leucocytosis, and abdominal pain. The clinical picture may be indistinguishable from acute appendicitis. Often the final diagnosis is made at laparotomy, when characteristic findings indicate Crohn disease.

Diverticulitis is high on the list of differential diagnoses, especially when the patient has a known history of diverticulosis. Fever, acute onset of abdominal pain, and leucocytosis are consistent with diverticulitis. However, the location of diverticulitis is typically in the left lower quadrant. In the case of redundant sigmoid colon, however, the pain can be located in the right lower quadrant. Diarrhea is often present in diverticulitis.

Colon cancer would not present in this fashion, and her abdominal pain with the CT findings does not support viral gastroenteritis.

Board Testing Point: Recognize the clinical features of acute appendicitis.

34. Answer: E

Answer: Abdominal CT scan.
She has known history of diverticulitis, and now with the findings of rebound tenderness and involuntary abdominal rigidity, there is the possibility of an abscess or perforation of a diverticulum. Emergent CT scan (or ultrasound) should be done to evaluate for this possibility. Colonoscopy and barium enema should be avoided during the active stage. If an abscess is found, drainage is necessary either with radiologic guidance or surgical intervention. Bowel rest is indicated, but you must rule out the possibility of something more severe such as abscess or perforation. A bleeding scan is not indicated since she has no evidence of a severe bleed.

Board Testing Point: Recognize the clinical features of diverticular disease with possible abscess/perforation complication.

35. Answer: A

Answer: Bright red blood on toilet paper in a 25-year-old man.
The 25-year-old man likely has hemorrhoids. Everyone needs a colonoscopy.

Board Testing Point: Recognize which clinical events would warrant colonoscopy for workup.

36. Answer: D

Answer: Arteriogram.
He has the findings of intestinal angina, also known as chronic mesenteric ischemia. He has the classic triad: abdominal pain after meals, abdominal bruit, and weight loss (from tolerating only small meals). Additionally, he smokes and has evidence of peripheral vascular disease (lower extremity findings). He needs an arteriogram to confirm evidence of occlusion in the splanchnic (intestinal) arteries. Treatment is with surgical bypass.

Board Testing Point: Recognize the clinical features of chronic mesenteric ischemia.

37. Answer: D

Answer: Hemoperitoneum.
He has now developed Cullen sign, which indicates the possibility of a hemoperitoneum. This means that severe necrotizing pancreatitis has developed.

Board Testing Point: Recognize the clinical significance of Cullen sign.

38. Answer: D

Answer: He has acute hepatitis B and past infection with A.
He has acute hepatitis B (he is in the "window" period). He has IgM antibody only to hepatitis B core. He has lost his HBsAg but not developed IgG antibody to hepatitis B core—commonly known as the "window" period. He also has IgG to hepatitis A, which means that he has had an old infection from which he recovered. There is no such thing as "chronic hepatitis A."

On most "screens" for hepatitis, do the following tests:

- Anti-HAV IgM—looks for acute hepatitis A
- HBsAg—looks for acute infection as well as chronic carrier states
- Anti-HBc IgM—looks for acute infection in the "window"
- Anti-HBc IgG—tells you if a person has been infected with hepatitis B in the past; does not tell you if he is still infectious; this requires the HBsAg test
- Hepatitis C antibody—this just tells you if someone has been infected with hepatitis C; it doesn't tell you status of infection (i.e., chronic infected or resolved)

Regarding the other options:

1) Acute hepatitis A and past infection with hepatitis B: Anti-HAV IgM positive; all of the hepatitis B tests are negative except hepatitis B core IgG antibody.
2) Chronic A and acute B: Impossible; remember that chronic A does not exist.
3) Chronic A and chronic B: Again, impossible.
4) Neither hepatitis A or hepatitis B: This would be correct if all the antibody studies were negative.

Board Testing Point: Know how to interpret hepatitis serologic tests.

---

39. Answer: D

Answer: Wilson disease.
The picture is showing you classic Kayser-Fleischer rings, the yellowish-brown discoloration in the cornea close to the limbus. It can present in many ways, but a chronic hepatitis-like picture is common. Multiple organs can be involved due to the excess amount of copper. This is an autosomal recessive disorder of copper metabolism. A mutated copper transporting enzyme prevents the excretion of copper detached from the copper-transporting ceruloplasmin into the bile. Rising copper levels inhibit ceruloplasmin formation from apo-ceruloplasmin. A marker for this disease is a low ceruloplasmin, but remember that the low ceruloplasmin does **not** cause the disease process; it is the excess copper. By the way, the Smith-Jones syndrome does not exist.

Board Testing Point: Recognize the clinical features of Wilson disease.

---

40. Answer: A

Answer: Percutaneous endoscopic gastrostomy (PEG) is appropriate intervention to allow hydration and nutrition.
This patient has oropharyngeal dysphagia, of which the most common cause is a CVA. There are other neurological causes as well, like ALS. The best study for this is the modified barium swallow. Endoscopy is not helpful at all in determining the reason for this type of dysphagia. PEG is considered a surgical procedure, and antibiotics do reduce the risk of infection afterwards. Other complications would include bowel perforation, bleeding and local cellulitis. Many patients will still aspirate after the procedure, although this is more commonly due to aspiration of saliva rather than reflux and aspiration of gastric contents.

Board Testing Point: Recognize the clinical utility of a percutaneous endoscopic gastrostomy in a patient who has had a recent cerebrovascular event.

---

41. Answer: A

Answer: Omeprazole 20 mg PO, before breakfast.
This patient appropriately underwent endoscopy because of his long history of reflux symptoms. Endoscopy is done to make sure there is no presence of Barrett esophagus, which in this case there was not. He does have significant esophagitis, and the issue is what type of treatment gives the most complete acid suppression. Proton pump inhibitors are stronger than the H2 receptor antagonist. However, to fully reach their potential, they should be given before a meal and after a fast—thus, before breakfast is the best time. When given in this way, the proton pump inhibitor will usually suppress acid production for 12–24 hours. The vast majority of patients with gross esophagitis will be found to completely heal with PPI therapy. Sucralfate has not been shown to have significant value in the treatment of reflux esophagitis.

Board Testing Point: Recognize that before breakfast is the best time to recommend taking proton pump inhibitors in the treatment of esophagitis.

42. Answer: D

Answer: Reflux esophagitis.
Odynophagia usually relates to acute esophageal injury from medications (e.g., doxycycline), instrumentation (naso-gastric tubing) or infections like herpes or *Candida*. Very rarely would reflux esophagitis lead to odynophagia. The appearance described is most consistent with a herpetic infection. Most cases of herpes esophagitis in the otherwise competent host are due to re-activation of a late herpes infection rather than primary infection. These are often brought out by high doses of corticosteroids. Biopsies from the edge of the ulcer are helpful, and the tissue should be sent for culture and histology. These patients may respond even without antiviral therapy, especially if the steroids can be discontinued.

Board Testing Point: Recognize common causes of odynophagia in an ICU patient.

43. Answer: C

Answer: 24-hour ambulatory pH probe may reveal abnormal reflux even without typical reflux symptoms.
By definition, this patient's motility shows diffuse esophageal spasm, which is characterized by intermittent simultaneous contractions amid normal peristalsis. The upper endoscopy in this case was a very low-yield procedure and probably added little to the management of this patient. However, a 24-hour ambulatory pH probe may reveal that some cases of diffuse esophageal spasm are due to reflux, even if the patient does not have typical reflux symptoms. In these cases, the chest pain will resolve with aggressive treatment of the reflux. Some cases of diffuse esophageal spasm will have dysphagia with the chest pain. However, in this case, since there is no dysphagia, there is no reason to expect the dilatation would help. Probably the most important aspect of treatment is reassurance of the patient. Nitrates are poorly tolerated on a long-term basis for this presentation. There may be a role for use of calcium-channel antagonists, anti-spasm medicines, or tricyclic antidepressants.

Board Testing Point: Recognize that a 24-hour ambulatory pH probe is an effective means to diagnose reflux, which may contribute to diffuse esophageal spasm.

44. Answer: C

Answer: Stomach.
Carcinoid rarely affects the stomach.

Board Testing Point: Recognize that carcinoid affects the GI tract but rarely affects the stomach.

45. Answer: A

Answer: Check the stool for *Clostridium difficile* toxin before initiating therapy.
This is a case of ulcerative colitis that has developed a secondary *Clostridium difficile* infection. Many flares of disease activity in patients with inflammatory bowel disease may be due to *Clostridium difficile*, and this needs to be aggressively considered. In the appropriate setting, the presence of fecal leukocytes would be good evidence of *C. difficile* infection—for instance, in the hospitalized patient who develops diarrhea after antibiotics. However, in the patient with IBD, who may have fecal leukocytes just related to their disease process, this would not be a reliable sign. Many patients, like the one described, will have a leukocytosis associated with *C. difficile*, although this is not specific. Flexible sigmoidoscopy may reveal pseudo-membranes but is not always diagnostic. Some patients do not have the characteristic pseudo-membranous colitis, and in some patients it may be located beyond the range of the flexible sigmoidoscope. In the patient with suspected *C. difficile* colitis, the stool should be sent (preferably 3 specimens) for *C. difficile* toxin. One does not need to send this stool for culture of *C. difficile*. The appropriate therapy is oral metronidazole.

Board Testing Point: Recognize that ulcerative colitis patients may become infected with *Clostridium difficile.*

46. Answer: B

Answer: Amoxicillin-clavulanate 875 mg PO bid.
This is a patient who has scleroderma and related bacterial overgrowth syndrome. Scleroderma has a wide variety of effects in the gastrointestinal tract. These patients often have severe esophageal disease because of the decreased esophageal peristalsis and the decreased lower esophageal sphincter tone. This leads to severe reflux complications like esophageal stricture and Barrett esophagus. Decreased gastric peristalsis is also seen. The wide-mouthed small bowel diverticula are characteristic of scleroderma, and the bacterial overgrowth is related to not only the diverticula, but also to poor peristalsis in the small bowel. The bacteria impair carbohydrate metabolism, which increases bowel distention. Vitamin deficiency is common in general, although the bacteria can produce Vitamin K, so it's rare to have a coagulopathy secondary to Vitamin K deficiency. The treatment is with broad-spectrum antibiotics. Many different treatments are available, including:

1) Rifamixin
2) Amoxicillin-clavulanate (expensive)
3) Metronidazole combined with:
   - Cephalosporin
   - TMP/SMX, or
   - Oral gentamicin
4) Norfloxacin

Erythromycin and azithromycin would not be awnticipated to help this patient and may even make the diarrhea worse. Metoclopramide might improve her gastric emptying, although this is not causing any symptoms at this time.

Board Testing Point: Recognize the clinical features of bacterial overgrowth syndrome.

47. Answer: A

Answer: By attaching a polyethylene glycol moiety to interferon alpha, there is an increased response rate. Interferon-alpha 2a had been the standard therapy for chronic hepatitis C, but treatment had been hampered by its short half-life and wide fluctuations in plasma concentration. A combination of interferon with ribavirin had been shown to have improved results. Likewise, a study demonstrating that PEG interferon-alpha 2a (which is the attachment of a polyethylene glycol moiety to the interferon molecule) causes improved results. When compared to standard interferon, the pegylated interferon had a virologic response at 48 weeks of 69% compared to 28% with interferon alone. Likewise, there was also improvement in the sustained normalization of ALT even at 72 weeks (45% vs 25%). Neutropenia and thrombocytopenia can occasionally complicate the treatment of hepatitis with interferon, but it would be uncommon for this to require cessation of therapy. The most common serious adverse effects are psychiatric, including severe depression. Factors that would predict a good response to interferon therapy include lower levels of HCV RNA and an HCV genotype other than Type 1.

Board Testing Point: Recognize the clinical features associated with a better virologic response to pegylated interferon in hepatitis C therapy.

48. Answer: B

Answer: Paracentesis is the appropriate diagnostic test at this time.
Spontaneous bacterial peritonitis is a potentially serious complication of any patient with ascites. Although it is most commonly seen with ascites due to cirrhosis, it can occur when the ascites is due to other causes as well. It may present with abdominal pain, fever, and hepatic encephalopathy, although not all of these symptoms are necessary. The patient may have neither pain nor fever. The risk factors for developing spontaneous bacterial peritonitis include:

- Prior episodes of SBP
- Bilirubin greater than 2.5
- Fluid protein level less than 1 g/dL
- Upper GI hemorrhage is also felt to be a risk factor for SBP, and empiric antibiotics are felt to have some prophylactic value.

The majority of episodes of SBP are due to enteric gram-negative bacteria and non-enterococcal *Streptococcus*. When performing paracentesis, one should inoculate the fluid directly into culture bottles, both aerobic and anaerobic, at the bedside. An absolute PMN count of greater than 250 confirms SBP. The most appropriate antimicrobial therapy would be cefotaxime 2 g IV q 6–12 hours. The aminoglycosides demonstrate significant toxicity in cirrhotic patients.

Board Testing Point: Recognize spontaneous bacterial peritonitis and that paracentesis is the best diagnostic test, as well as cefotaxime as appropriate treatment.

49. Answer: C

Answer: Transferrin saturation greater than 50% should prompt further evaluation, including HFE gene determination.

Hereditary hemochromatosis is a common inherited disorder with a prevalence of 1 in 200 to 1 in 400 in populations of northern European descent. It has autosomal recessive pattern of inheritance, and the gene for the disease, known as the HFE, has recently been discovered. The patients may present with fatigue, malaise, abdominal pain, arthralgias, and impotence. However, if discovered by screening of family members or screening of asymptomatic individuals, the majority have no complications such as cirrhosis. Physical examination of patients with hemochromatosis may reveal hepatomegaly and skin hyperpigmentation. Serum iron is generally elevated, and the iron saturation is greater than 50%. Values such as these should prompt further gene testing. The serum ferritin is usually abnormal, but can be abnormal in other diseases, such as alcoholic liver disease and HCV. If this patient is found to have hereditary hemochromatosis by genetic testing, then he should undergo weekly therapeutic phlebotomy of 500 mL of whole blood until his transferrin saturation is less than 50% and the serum ferritin is less than 50 mg/L.

Board Testing Point: Recognize the clinical features of hemochromatosis and when further diagnostic testing is appropriate.

50. Answer: D

Answer: Drug hepatotoxicity.

If one includes acetaminophen, then drug hepatotoxicity is clearly the most common cause of acute liver failure in the United States. Acetaminophen is the single most important causative agent, although many other drugs may cause this as well. In cases of acetaminophen hepatotoxicity, many are due to suicide attempts. However, there are many others who have this due to accidental toxicity during attempts at pain relief. This can occur if the person over several days is ingesting relatively large doses of acetaminophen. Alcoholics seem to be at risk for toxicity even at lower than usual levels of acetaminophen ingestion. Suicide patients often present promptly, but the accidental toxicity patient may have a delayed presentation, and therefore often has higher mortality. If the patient does present early on, then N-acetyl-cystine may be helpful if administered promptly. Some cases do progress to absolute liver failure, which would require transplantation.

Board Testing Point: Recognize that drug toxicity is the most common cause of liver failure in the U.S.

51. Answer: A

Answer: Upper GI small bowel series.

This is a 55-year-old with occult GI bleeding that has been severe enough to cause profound anemia requiring blood transfusions. No source was found for the bleeding in either the upper or the lower tract. Likely, this is due to a small bowel bleeding source. Although it is possible that this could be due to an AV malformation, which is the most common source of small bowel bleeding, he is younger than most patients with this type of bleeding. Therefore, one thinks of other possibilities, which includes tumors of the small bowel, which can present with bleeding. For this indication, one could do either an enteroscopy or an upper GI small bowel series. The x-ray has the advantage of visualizing the entire bowel, although it's not as accurate for the upper region of the jejunum as enteroscopy would be. It is controversial whether estrogen would have helped AV malformation bleeding anyway, and this medicine is very poorly tolerated in men. There is no indication that bleeding rate is rapid enough for a tagged RBC scan to be beneficial. If the GI series demonstrates a tumor in the small bowel, then a CT scan would be appropriate, but not at this point.

Board Testing Point: Recognize that workup of occult GI bleed after upper endoscopy and colonoscopy includes small bowel series.

52. Answer: D

Answer: Start patient on iron and monitor the Hgb every 2 months.
This gentleman likely was bleeding from the AVM found in the cecum. The diverticulosis that was found was not the cause of the bleeding, because this does not cause occult bleeding. Diverticular bleeding generally cause an acute bleed with significant hemorrhage, resulting in maroon stool. Likewise, the polyp is too small to cause any bleeding. However, even though the AVM was the likely cause of bleeding, at this point it has not resulted in significant blood loss such that the patient is symptomatic. It is likely that this patient can be placed on iron and his Hgb will stabilize. He may slowly ooze blood from time to time, but the iron will replace those losses. Estrogen therapy is not of proven value for AV malformations, and it's not tolerated by men because of the side effects. H_2 blockers are not indicated in AVM treatment.

Board Testing Point: Recognize that iron therapy is appropriate in a patient who presents with iron deficiency from an AVM without overt bleeding.

53. Answer: C

Answer: This patient will likely not have recurrent bleeding after admission, though his HCT will likely fall with hydration.
This patient does have bleeding from a Mallory-Weiss tear, and it is often the case that the patient does not remember prior retching. However, given that there is no fresh blood in the stomach, no oozing from the linear tear, or visible vessel, he does have a favorable prognosis in that the bleeding has likely stopped. There is no indication for endoscopic therapy unless there is active bleeding or a visible vessel. Mallory-Weiss tears can certainly be a cause of massive hemorrhage, although not in this case.

Board Testing Point: Recognize favorable prognosis factors in a patient with a Mallory-Weiss tear.

54. Answer: A

Answer: Discharge home on lansoprazole 30 mg qd with caution to return to the emergency department in case of another black stool.
This patient has developed a duodenal ulcer, probably due to the daily aspirin intake. However, the bleeding stopped several days ago and with the endoscopic picture showing a clean base, there is very little likelihood of further bleeding. Her risk of rebleeding at this point is between 0 and 5%. At this point, it is very safe to let her go home on oral therapy for the ulcer. She needs to be advised to avoid aspirin. There is no value to endoscopic treatment in this patient, which would be indicated only if there were a visible vessel or active bleeding.

Board Testing Point: Recognize the prognostic value of a "clean base" in a patient with a duodenal ulcer.

55. Answer: C

Answer: Colonoscopy and endoscopy. If the latter is grossly normal, obtain oriented biopsies of the duodenum.

The patient has celiac disease. This has led to the bloating and loose stools, which represent malabsorption, as well as her iron deficiency anemia. The iron deficiency anemia may not be due to occult bleeding, but rather interference with the absorption of iron, which takes place mainly in the duodenum. The duodenum is the region in the small bowel most affected by celiac disease, and it is not uncommon for these patients to be iron-deficient. However, performing a colonoscopy and endoscopy is correct because in her age group, a full endoscopic evaluation needs to be done on anybody with an iron deficiency anemia, even in the absence of heme-positive stools. Clearly, colonoscopy needs to be done to rule out colon cancer. On upper exam, there are some characteristic findings that can indicate celiac disease. The duodenal folds may be atrophic or have a scalloped appearance. However, even in the absence of endoscopic findings, one should do the oriented biopsies of the duodenum if one suspects celiac disease. The upper GI series would not be accurate enough to show any specific changes for celiac disease. The antigliadin and antiendomysial antibodies can be helpful in diagnosing patients with celiac disease, but today the best test is either IgA (not IgG) antiendomysial antibody or tissue transglutaminase (tTG) antibody. The antigliadin antibody is non-specific. Also the gold standard of diagnosis stills relies on duodenal biopsies, and one should have that before making the diagnosis and initiating therapy. Additionally, steroids are not indicated at this time. In this case, one would simply treat with a gluten-free diet.

Board Testing Point: Recognize the clinical features of celiac disease and how to diagnose/work up a patient with classic findings.

---

56. Answer: B

Answer: ERCP.

This patient with ulcerative colitis has likely developed primary sclerosing cholangitis. Of all patients with PSC, 70% will have a history of ulcerative colitis. As in the case of this patient, there is a strong male predominance. Many of these patients are asymptomatic at the onset. Some will give symptoms of cholangitis, such as fever and chills, and some may present with fatigue and malaise. At the time of ERCP, there may be multiple strictures of both the intra and extrahepatic bile ducts. There often is not enough dilatation for this to be noted on studies such as the ultrasound. Dominant strictures of the bile duct can be dilated at the time of ERCP. There is no additional value to a liver biopsy at this time. An abdominal CT scan would likely not add any more than the ultrasound already did. And finally, there is no indication for laparoscopic cholecystectomy either.

Board Testing Point: Recognize the association of primary sclerosing cholangitis in a patient with ulcerative colitis and that an ERCP is indicated.

---

57. Answer: A

Answer: ERCP now, since there is a high likelihood of stones present in the CBD.
This woman has had a case of pancreatitis likely secondary to a passed gallstone. Although the ultrasound did not show any stone or stones in the common duct or dilatation in the common duct, there are several factors here that would predict a moderate possibility of persistent stones in the duct. This would be the fact that her laboratories increased on the day after admission and that her bilirubin went as high as 3.5. Therefore, with this moderate possibility of retained stones in the CBD, an ERCP is reasonable. ERCP does not necessarily have to be done before cholecystectomy. Some would say do a laparoscopic cholecystectomy with an intraoperative cholangiogram, and then proceed with an ERCP after surgery if the cholangiogram is positive for stones. However, this is a case where it is probably appropriate to do the study preoperatively. There is no value in sending the patient home before coming back to have surgery in this case, since her abdomen is completely benign. Likewise, there is no reason why she can't have a laparoscopic cholecystectomy, and there is no need for the increased morbidity associated with the open procedure with common duct exploration. Although percutaneous cholangiogram will clearly identify stones in the common duct, it does not have the same therapeutic potential of being able to remove the stones readily that an ERCP does.

Board Testing Point: Recognize laboratory and imaging abnormalities that would suggest biliary pancreatitis.

58. Answer: C

Answer: Consult surgery for elective resection of the tail of the pancreas with removal of the cyst.
This patient does indeed have a cyst in the pancreas, but it is unlikely that this is a pseudocyst, given that she has never had pain or symptoms to suggest either acute or chronic pancreatitis. In this case, one must consider the possibility of a cystic neoplasm, which can be either a cystadenoma or a cystadenocarcinoma or, rarely, cystic islet cell tumors. A CA19-9 level might be elevated in cases of pancreatic adenocarcinoma, but it would not be helpful in the cystic neoplasms. Likewise, CT-directed needle aspiration often yields negative cytology even in the case of cystadenocarcinoma. Since this woman is healthy, she should undergo resection of the tail of the pancreas, which is a relatively easy procedure and will be curative in this case.

Board Testing Point: Recognize the clinical features and treatment of a cystic neoplasm in a patient with a pancreatic cyst.

59. Answer: B

Answer: This is likely a *Staphylococcus aureus* food poisoning.
These patients have the typical description of *Staph aureus* food poisoning. Patients usually present 4–6 hours after ingestion of the food with nausea, vomiting, and diarrhea. These symptoms do not last long, rarely more than 12 hours, but it is not uncommon to have severe dehydration. The *Staph aureus* could have been obtained in the ham or even the deviled eggs. Although undercooked poultry can be a source of *Salmonella*, the incubation period is much longer than what is seen here. Likewise, in *E. coli* O157, the incubation period is longer as well. Giardiasis can occur after ingesting Rocky Mountain water, but the symptoms are too severe in this case and the timing is too soon after the picnic.

The treatment of *Staph aureus* food poisoning revolves around supportive intravenous fluid. This is an ingested toxin rather than an active bacteria, so there is no value in giving antibiotics.

Board Testing Point: Recognize the clinical features of *Staphylococcus aureus* food poisoning.

60. Answer: D

Answer: Small bowel resection.
Small bowel resections are common in the setting of necrotic appendicitis. Though resections of more than several centimeters are less common, they do happen on occasion. The terminal ileum is the only place where vitamin B_{12} is resorbed as well as conjugated bile acids. When > 2 feet of the terminal ileum is resected, bile acid diarrhea and B_{12} deficiency result. This patient's diarrhea plus B_{12} deficiency suggest a malabsorption problem. Atrophic gastritis also causes B_{12} deficiency but is less likely in this setting since no history was given to suggest it as a cause. Crohn ileitis is associated strongly with B_{12} deficiency, but the ESR and CRP are normal. HIV is another cause of B_{12} deficiency, but wouldn't be suspected with this patient's history.

Board Testing Point: Know the causes of B_{12} deficiency and macrocytic anemia.

61. Answer: B

Answer: 3–5 years from his last endoscopy.
There are variety of guidelines and consensus statements regarding Barrett esophagus. Typically the guidelines agree that for no dysplasia, surveillance endoscopies with biopsies should be done every 3–5 years. With low-grade dysplasia, every 6–12 months, and with high-grade dysplasia and no therapy, every 3 months.

Board Testing Point: Be generally familiar with the cancer screening guidelines for patients with Barrett esophagus.

62. Answer: B

Answer: Colonoscopy now and then annual colonoscopy.
This patient has primary sclerosing cholangitis (PSC) and UC and therefore has a very high risk for colon cancer—up to 25%. He has not had a complete colonoscopy, only a flexible sigmoidoscopy. Patients diagnosed with UC and PSC need a full colonoscopy with surveillance biopsies at the time of diagnosis and annually for the rest of their lives.

Board Testing Point: Know the findings that indicate PSC. Know of increased cancer risk and need for annual colonoscopy in a patient with both PSC and UC.

63. Answer: C

Answer: Order a CT of the abdomen.
This patient has the hallmarks of chronic pancreatitis—weight loss and severe steatorrhea. Confirmatory tests:

- CT of the abdomen has an 85% sensitivity (showing pancreatic atrophy, calcifications, or a dilated pancreatic duct) and is the initial procedure of choice in diagnosing chronic pancreatis.
- Endoscopic ultrasound, done by a skilled gastroenterologist, is the procedure of choice in some centers.
- An abdominal x-ray showing calcifications (30% sensitivity) is also confirmatory.
- Abdominal ultrasound can also be used.
- MRCP can also be used but is usually a follow-up test in patients with negative initial tests.
- ERCP is largely a therapeutic, rather than a diagnostic, intervention.

Placing the patient on pancreatic enzymes without imaging the pancreas first is not a good idea because she could have some other cause of malabsorption. The carboxylate-deficient transferrin test is used to help detect heavy alcohol use. While alcohol could cause some mild malabsorption, it wouldn't cause the severe steatorrhea she currently has.

Board Testing Point: Recognize the presentation of chronic pancreatitis and the confirmatory tests.

64. Answer: B

Answer: Adenocarcinoma of the esophagus.
This patient likely has an esophageal adenocarcinoma since the lesion is in the distal 1/3 of the esophagus. Squamous cell carcinoma usually occurs in the proximal esophagus. While esophageal hematomas are described in patients on anticoagulants, the long history of dysphagia in this case argues against an etiology of this esophageal filling defect. A food bezoar in the esophagus would not present with a radiograph showing a luminal narrowing and filling defect.

Board Testing Point: Know what types of cancer tend to appear in different regions of the esophagus.

65. Answer: B

Answer: Referral for Nissen fundoplication.
This patient would be a good candidate for a Nissen fundoplication, because she has responded well to PPI medications—this is the single best indicator of success. Repeat EGD now would not be helpful. This patient had erosive esophagitis on a prior endoscopy and has an 80% chance of recurrence of severe reflux symptoms off of PPI. Metoclopramide was used as a reflux/heartburn treatment in the past but is limited in use in 2014 because of side effects.

Board Testing Point: Know when Nissen fundoplication is considered in a patient with GERD.

66. Answer: B

Answer: Barium swallow.
The barium swallow is often the 1st test performed in the workup of esophageal dysphagia, unless the etiology is known from past evaluations. Some experts do EGD first, but barium swallow is definitely done as the 1st test if symptoms are severe or if there is new-onset dysphagia with liquids, because it can reveal functional components that endoscopy cannot find.

Barium swallow is especially done before endoscopy for the following reasons:

- There is a risk of perforation when endoscoping a patient with diverticula or high-grade obstruction.
- Information from the barium swallow may preclude the need for endoscopy.
- Information from the barium swallow provides the endoscopist a general idea of the type and severity of the underlying lesion.
- The patient is high risk is at high risk for sedation-related complications.

This patient with severe CAD and dementia is at high risk for endoscopy and procedural sedation. Sometimes a barium swallow is done after a negative EGD to rule out lower esophageal rings or external compression that can be missed with EGD. Chest CT is of limited utility in working up intermittent dysphagia. Modified barium swallow study is an evaluation of the upper esophagus and would not be helpful here.

Board Testing Point: Know the indications for barium swallow vs. EGD.

67. Answer: D

Answer: Right upper quadrant ultrasound.
Remember that alcoholic hepatitis is clinically indistinguishable from ascending cholangitis. This patient has the entire classic "Charcot triad" of findings: RUQ pain, jaundice, and fever. An obstructing common bile duct stone needs to be ruled out before starting treatment for alcoholic hepatitis. ERCP is the preferred therapeutic maneuver once a diagnosis of an obstructing stone is made, but it is not a diagnostic test. MRCP is an option, but this patient is unstable, and an ultrasound is usually sufficient for diagnosis.

Board Testing Point: Know what test to do to differentiate alcoholic hepatitis from ascending cholangitis.

68. Answer: C

Answer: 24-hour urinary 5HIAA and serum chromogranin.
These symptoms are especially prominent in hormone-secreting carcinoids; the initial evaluation should include a check for increased urinary excretion of 5-hydroxyindoleacetic acid (5-HIAA) and serum chromogranin A level.

The bone marrow biopsy and FLIP1-PDGFRα indicate the workup and diagnosis of hypereosinophilic syndrome, but there is no eosinophilia in the peripheral blood and, hence, these 2 tests are not required. The TEE options are aimed at ruling out infective endocarditis, which can also cause new onset murmurs, but there are no signs of infection. Hence, this clinical scenario is aimed at recognizing the carcinoid syndrome.

Board Testing Point: Recognize carcinoid and its complications.

69. Answer: A

Answer: FNA of the lymph node and GI colonoscopy and/or endoscopy.
A left supraclavicular lymph node that is solitary and hard is called "Virchow node" or Troisier sign. It is suspicious for metastatic GI cancer. The labs also suggest iron deficiency anemia, and upper GI malignancy, like gastric cancer, is top in the differential. Management of iron deficiency anemia in a male > 50 years of age entails ruling out blood loss from the GI tract.

Although lymphoma can present with supraclavicular lymphadenopathy, it is unlikely to be lymphoma due to the fact that this is a single node, with hard consistency. And, again, the iron deficiency anemia is more likely caused by chronic GI bleeding from cancer.

Board Testing Point: Recognize suspicious signs of GI malignancy and follow up with the appropriate workup.

70. Answer: C

Answer: Refer for genetic testing, colonoscopy, U/A, and gynecologic exam.
Lynch syndrome is the result of an autosomal dominant mutation of a mismatch repair gene that causes increased tendency to have a variety of cancers within a family line, especially colon and uterine cancer. This patient meets the rather nonsensitive Amsterdam II criteria for Lynch syndrome, which is ≥ 3 relatives over at least 2 generations with 1 person being < 50 years old (the 3-2-1 rule). She also has rectal bleeding, which is longstanding and merits workup. Surveillance colonoscopy every 1–2 years is recommended as cancer screening for Lynch syndrome, but other testing is required in the initial workup for the diagnosis, which includes ruling out colon and uterine cancer in women. Ultimately genetic testing is done on the patient and, if positive, other family members will undergo genetic counseling. EGD is not one of those tests.

Board Testing Point: Know the clinical criteria and basic workup for Lynch syndrome.

PULMONARY MEDICINE

71. Answer: E

Answer: Start enteral feeding.
Enteral feeds are preferred over TPN because enteral feeds will maintain the intestinal epithelium and its natural defenses against bacteria. There is no reason to make this patient NPO.

Board Testing Point: Recognize the need for adequate nutrition in a patient who requires prolonged mechanical ventilation.

72. Answer: E

Answer: CT of chest to evaluate the nodule.
Calcified nodules are usually benign; however, increasing evidence has shown that almost all nodules need an initial CT scan. Then if things look OK, serial CT scans to follow up. Even though this patient is low-risk and this is likely old histoplasmosis, it warrants workup. This has been a change in thinking with the goal being not to miss any resectable lung cancers. For this patient, if the 5-mm nodule appears to be consistent with a benign lesion, repeat CT would be done in 6 to 12 months; if this shows no change, then it would be safe to stop surveillance. If changed, resection is warranted. Of note is that if he had a "popcorn" calcified pattern, this likely would be a hamartoma, but you would still check a CT scan and follow as indicated to be sure. Solitary nodules **without** calcifications are also watched with serial CT scans. If the patient is higher-risk (smoker, family history, etc.), these scans may be repeated in 3 months if the initial scan appears non-cancerous. Many would just proceed with excision, particularly if there are suspicions of malignancy.

Board Testing Point: Know how to work up an isolated pulmonary nodule.

73. Answer: A

Answer: Bronchoalveolar lavage and/or transbronchial lung biopsy.
This patient has an interstitial lung disease with restricted lung volumes and a reduced diffusing capacity; and it will worsen without definitive diagnosis and treatment. Serial PFTs would merely provide confirmation of what you already suspect. You need to know which ILD the patient has and how to stage it in terms of activity to decide on treatment options. Most would begin with bronchoalveolar lavage with transbronchial lung biopsy. If this is negative, then a high-resolution CT could be performed, or some would just proceed to the definitive open lung biopsy. The yield on transbronchial biopsy is very good for some etiologies (particularly sarcoid or infectious etiologies). However, in order to provide an adequate tissue sample for examination, an open-lung biopsy (traditional or thorascopic) is often required. This is not consistent with pulmonary embolism, and V-Q scanning or CT angiography are not indicated. Open-lung biopsy certainly could be considered, but you would not resect all of the areas of "diseased lung" without a known diagnosis or reason.

Board Testing Point: Know how to work up interstitial lung disease.

74. Answer: B

Answer: Carbon monoxide poisoning.
All of the workers were diagnosed as suffering from carbon monoxide poisoning. CO has been called the silent killer and is the cause of approximately 5,000 deaths annually, with 2 to 5 times that number requiring treatment. Even with treatment, the devastating sequelae that can accompany CO poisoning can be life-changing. These include chorea, rigidity, dementia, myoclonus, impaired sensory function, seizures, and gait dysfunction. There can also be permanent cardiac damage due to the hypoxia involved in the poisoning process.

CO is an odorless, colorless, and tasteless gas that results from incomplete combustion of fuels (i.e., coal, wood, gasoline). Once inhaled, it binds quickly and tightly to the hemoglobin (Hgb) and crowds out the oxygen; studies have shown CO can bind 200 times stronger than oxygen. Since the Hgb can no longer carry the oxygen, the patient becomes hypoxemic and anoxic. Also, the CO binds with myoglobin in the muscles and interferes with cellular metabolism, causing metabolic acidosis.

Normal carboxyhemoglobin (HbCO) levels are 0–3% for nonsmokers and 3–8% for smokers. A level of 10–20% causes headaches, nausea, vomiting, and dyspnea. A level of 30–40% causes severe headaches, syncope, and tachyarrhythmias. Levels greater than 40% cause Cheyne-Stokes respiration or respiratory failure, seizures, unconsciousness, permanent brain damage, cardiac arrest, and even death.

Because of the vagueness of the symptoms and their similarity to flu-like symptoms (nausea, vomiting, dizziness, headache, etc.), CO poisoning is often misdiagnosed. Also, even if HbCO is present, it cannot be diagnosed with a simple pulse oximetry device—because the displayed saturation level equals the sum of the oxyhemoglobin and carboxyhemoglobin.

So if you suspect a patient has CO poisoning, what should you do? First and foremost, the patient needs high-flow, high-concentration O_2, preferably a non-rebreather mask at 15 liters per minute, as well as a large bore IV. Prepare for blood draws (ABG, CBC, electrolytes, CPK, lactate, and carboxyhemoglobin). A urine sample is also useful to rule out rhabdomyolysis (cardiac muscle breakdown secondary to the myoglobin damage from CO). Other treatment modalities may include a CXR, cardiac monitoring, and possibly mannitol to help decrease the cerebral edema accompanying the CO poisoning. Finally, probably the most effective treatment is transfer of the patient to a hyperbaric oxygen unit (HBO). This is clearly indicated when the patient is very symptomatic and/or the HbCO is 25% or greater.

Board Testing Point: Recognize the clinical features of carbon monoxide poisoning.

75. Answer: D

Answer: Ciprofloxacin.
The problem is that he is on theophylline and adding ciprofloxacin has caused his theophylline clearance to decrease, thus resulting in increased serum levels of theophylline. The result of increased theophylline levels in the toxic range usually begins with nausea and vomiting. The other antibiotics listed do not induce changes in theophylline clearance.

Board Testing Point: Recognize the drug-drug interaction between ciprofloxacin and theophylline.

76. Answer: D

Answer: Low rate, small tidal volume, high flows.
When ventilating an asthmatic patient, the idea of "permissive hypercapnia" is important to remember. Focus on getting the oxygen saturation up and don't worry as much about the pCO_2. Each of the factors (low rate, small tidal volume, high flows) addresses the need for a prolonged expiratory phase. High flow on the inspiration allows for less time devoted to inspiration and more time to expiration. So based on the idea of "permissive hypercapnia," it makes sense to have a lower rate and smaller tidal volume.

Board Testing Point: Recognize how to ventilate a patient with asthma.

77. Answer: C

Answer: Supplemental oxygen should be worn 24 hours a day by this patient.
Only objective data from an arterial blood gas is acceptable to Medicare for supplemental oxygen. History and physical examination will not help get this funded. He needs to meet one of the following criteria:

1. Resting $P_aO_2 \leq 55$ mmHg, **or**
2. O_2 saturation $\leq 88\%$, **or**
3. $P_aO_2 \leq 59$ mmHg (O_2 sat $\leq 89\%$) with evidence of cor pulmonale

Evidence of cor pulmonale in these considerations is:

- Clinical evidence of right heart failure
- Pulmonale on ECG (p wave height > 2.5 mm in II, III, and AVF
- Hct > 55.6 (due to polycythemia from chroinic hypoxia 2° cor pulmonale)

You can tell him that being on supplemental oxygen is likely to improve his symptoms and there is a possibility that, in several months, he may not need the oxygen anymore. Medicare guidelines require you to bring him back between 61 and 90 days and retest him. Note that the use of supplemental oxygen does **not** depress the respiratory drive and cause an elevated CO_2. This is due to several factors, including an easing of pulmonary vasoconstriction, which leads to perfusion of previously underperfused spaces and possibly due to ventilation of previous dead space.

Board Testing Point: Know the Medicare criteria for home oxygen therapy.

78. Answer: D

Answer: Family history.
It would be exceedingly unusual for a male patient with cystic fibrosis to have children. The rest of the findings are consistent with CF. Remember that this gene is encoded on Chromosome 7. It causes a defect in sodium and chloride transport channels in lungs particularly, but also in other organs.

Board Testing Point: Recognize the clinical features associated with cystic fibrosis.

79. Answer: D

Answer: PEEP of 10 cm H_2O.
PEEP should be less than 5 cm H_2O before discontinuation of mechanical ventilation and extubation can be considered. Vital capacity should be greater than 10 to 15 mL/kg. Tidal volume of 4 to 5 mL/kg is acceptable for removal from the ventilator. FiO_2 should be less than 40% before discontinuation of mechanical ventilation. P(A-a) O_2 at an FiO_2 of 100%, less than 350 mmHg would also indicate increased probability of successful weaning off the ventilator and extubation.

Board Testing Point: Recognize the criteria for attempting to stop mechanical ventilation.

80. Answer: D

Answer: Start INH prophylaxis.
This patient has silicosis based on his history of working in a brickyard and the classic CXR findings of small nodules in the upper lobes that are calcified and the "hilar eggshell calcifications." There is no specific treatment for uncomplicated silicosis. The problem with silicosis, however, is that alveolar macrophages are made ineffective by the ingestion of silica; therefore, patients with silicosis are at increased risk of tuberculosis. Therefore, anytime a patient with known silicosis has a positive PPD, no matter what age or duration, he should be "prophylaxed" with INH. He has no evidence of active disease, and therefore treatment with 4-drug therapy is not indicated. Asbestosis more commonly involves the lower lobes, and his presentation does not warrant a big workup for this disease.

Board Testing Point: Recognize the increased risk of tuberculosis with a history of silicosis.

81. Answer: D

Answer: Langerhans cells.
This patient most likely has eosinophilic granuloma. Langerhans cells are the predominant cell form. It occurs in smokers and men much more often than in women. About 10% of patients will present with pneumothorax.

The diabetes insipidus is seen when the granuloma involve the posterior pituitary. Treatment is to **stop smoking**. If he had lytic bone lesions (particularly skull), diabetes insipidus, and exophthalmus, then he would have Hand-Schüller-Christian syndrome.

Board Testing Point: Recognize the association of Langerhans cells and eosinophilic granuloma.

82. Answer: A

Answer: Pulmonary sarcoidosis.
Her chest radiograph shows a diffuse miliary pattern, which is suspicious for tuberculous or metastatic carcinoma. Her biopsy shows 2 small, non-necrotizing granulomas. The differential diagnosis includes mainly infectious granulomatous disease, hypersensitivity pneumonia, and sarcoidosis. Granulomas may also be seen with aspiration pneumonia, in chronic beryllium disease, or exposure to titanium or aluminum dusts, as a response to certain drugs, and rarely with granulomatosis with polyangiitis (Wegener's), lymphocytic interstitial pneumonia or eosinophilic pneumonia. Tuberculosis has been effectively ruled out at this point, and bacterial pneumonia does

not fit this clinical picture or any of the results. Asbestosis would cause parenchymal fibrosis and involves lower lobes. The bronchoscopy findings are inconsistent with asbestosis. Granulomatosis with polyangiitis (Wegener's) is on the differential as mentioned above, but we have no evidence of renal disease, and it is much rarer than sarcoidosis in the African-American population.

Board Testing Point: Recognize the clinical features of sarcoidosis.

---

83. Answer: D

Answer: Restrictive ventilatory defect and marked decrease in diffusing capacity.
Note that FVC and FEV_1 are reduced in parallel—this suggests a restrictive ventilatory defect. The marked decrease in diffusing capacity suggests loss of capillary surface area, which may be seen in pulmonary fibrosis, emphysema, or pulmonary vascular disease.

Board Testing Point: Be able to interpret pulmonary function tests.

---

84. Answer: D

Answer: Cavitary rheumatoid nodules.
This man's major pulmonary findings were the cavitary rheumatoid nodules. Cancer and infection were excluded by histology and culture. Given the pattern of angiitis and granulomatosis (nodules), granulomatosis with polyangiitis (Wegener's) could not be excluded histologically. The lack of upper respiratory and renal abnormalities and the presence of known rheumatoid arthritis, in which similar histologic findings occur, favored the diagnosis of rheumatoid angiitis and nodules.

Board Testing Point: Be able to diagnose rheumatoid lung disease.

---

85. Answer: C

Answer: Pulmonary embolism.
There is an increased risk of thromboembolic disease during pregnancy with possible contributing factors including:

- Decreased vasomotor tone due to increased prostaglandins
- Venous compression by the gravid uterus
- Hypercoagulability due to increased levels of coagulation factors I, II, VIII, IX, and X
- Decreased plasma fibrinolytic activity

This patient had her onset of pulmonary embolism approximately 1 week ago. Thrombolytic therapy is as effective if started in 6–14 days as compared to within 5 days of pulmonary embolism.

Her ECG is classic. The S_1, Q3, T3 pattern is what is classically described but usually not seen. Echocardiogram is consistent with PE. With treatment and resolution, her tricuspid regurgitation disappeared. Her right ventricle also returned to normal size as did her pulmonary artery systolic pressure.

Board Testing Point: Recognize pulmonary embolism.

---

86. Answer: B

Answer: Fat embolism.
Based on the findings of dyspnea, confusion, and petechiae (particularly neck, conjunctiva, and axilla [not described in this patient]), you can make the diagnosis of fat emboli in the setting of a recent large bone fracture. Fat emboli can also occur after aggressive CPR and with sickle cell bone occlusive crisis. Treatment is supportive; unless the patient has secondary ARDS, steroids have **not** proven of benefit. We don't give you a lot of lab values here, and you shouldn't need them at this point. Again, the triad of dyspnea, confusion, and petechiae in the setting of recent fracture … think of fat embolism!

Board Testing Point: Be familiar with clinical scenarios that would produce fat embolism.

87. Answer: E

Answer: Admit to the hospital, place a chest tube, and start intravenous ceftriaxone and azithromycin.
He began with a community-acquired pneumonia and now has an empyema by definition: He has organisms seen on Gram stain of his pleural fluid! The organism is likely pneumococcus. Because he has an empyema, you must place the chest tube as soon as possible; he will not get better without drainage of the pus. Intravenous antibiotics alone will not work. Waiting 24 hours or consulting a pulmonologist will not change the basic fact that he needs "drano"! If you chose to send this patient home, you get 20 lashes with a wet noodle. Remember: Organisms on Gram stain of pleural fluid = **needs chest tube**. Finally, the choice of vancomycin and gentamicin for synergy is not correct. This choice would be useful if you thought he had community-acquired MRSA, for which he has no risk factors and his Gram stain is not consistent (you would expect gram-positive cocci in clusters for *Staphylococcus*).

Board Testing Point: Recognize and know how to treat empyema.

88. Answer: A

Answer: *Staphylococcus aureus.*
She recently had influenza, a classic setting where staphylococcal pneumonia will occur. *Streptococcus pneumoniae* is still very common in these patients also. Influenza virus is known to both increase respiratory colonization by *S. aureus* and impair ciliary function (and therefore clearance of staphylococci).

Board Testing Point: Recognize the association of recent influenza infection with *Staphylococcus aureus* pneumonia.

89. Answer: E

Answer: Continue current therapy.
Clinically she is doing well. You are weaning her off the vent; her physical examination is stable; her laboratory is stable (**<u>never</u> base antibiotic therapy** on a **minor bump in WBC**). The sputum results are not unusual for a patient in the Intensive Care Unit; they will frequently become colonized with gram-negative organisms—particularly *Pseudomonas*. Never change therapy based on just a tracheal aspirate; you must have some other change in exam or laboratory that is significant for you to consider treating the organism found on a tracheal aspirate.

Board Testing Point: Recognize that sputum results from a tracheal aspirate are rarely useful.

90. Answer: D

Answer: *Francisella tularensis.*
You need to put together the following: He is from Arkansas—if you see this state, think Blastomycosis, Histoplasmosis, Ehrlichiosis and Tularemia (a mnemonic for those of you mnemonically driven: BHET—Bill and Hillary Eat Toads in Arkansas). Second, he is a hunter in Arkansas: Say the 4 organisms again! Third, he has a pneumonia that is unresponsive to ceftriaxone—think of an unusual organism, which could be any of our 4 choices (BHET). Finally, they tell you that he is growing a gram-negative rod. Put Arkansas, pneumonia, and gram-negative rod together and there is only one choice: tularemia, which is caused by *Francisella tularensis*.

Board Testing Point: Recognize tularemia.

91. Answer: A

Answer: *Chlamydophila pneumoniae*
With the history of prior sore throat and now a febrile illness with documented pneumonia by chest x-ray, *Chlamydophila pneumoniae* is the most likely. The parrot is a red herring here because she had no signs of *C. psittaci* infection—look for a pneumonia with an extensive interstitial pattern that appears to be much worse than the physical exam would indicate. *C. trachomatis,* remember, causes genitourinary disease. *Staphylococcus aureus* would be seen after an influenza-like illness or if she were immunocompromised, and she would be much sicker. Don't be thrown by the positive throat culture for this organism—it can be found frequently in asymptomatic people. *H. influenzae* should not cause pneumonia in her age group.

Board Testing Point: Recognize the clinical features associated with *Chlamydophila pneumoniae* pneumonia.

92. Answer: C

Answer: Azithromycin 500 mg 2 PO today, then 1 PO q day x 4 days.
This patient could have *Streptococcus pneumoniae, Mycoplasma pneumoniae,* or *Chlamydophila pneumoniae*. Azithromycin and gatifloxacin are the only agents listed that are effective against all 3 organisms. The problem is that she is 17—note the ABIM will follow the FDA rules. You cannot give a quinolone to a child under the age of 18 except in special circumstances (anthrax, cystic fibrosis patients, etc.). The beta-lactam antibiotics listed are great for pneumococcus but won't get the atypicals. In an adolescent with uncomplicated pneumonia, look for a macrolide or doxycycline as an acceptable choice.

Board Testing Point: Know the treatment guidelines for community acquired pneumonia.

93. Answer: D

Answer: Start INH 300 mg daily for 9 months.
This nurse is a recent converter. He has had a 10 mm increase in 1 year's time. By definition, he should receive prophylaxis. His CXR is normal and he has no signs or symptoms of tuberculosis; therefore, he does not need to be treated for active tuberculosis. 12 months of INH is no longer recommended for anyone, including HIV-infected patients! It is not reasonable to repeat the PPD in 2 weeks; he has a positive result, and it will not change with repeated testing.

Board Testing Point: Know how to interpret PPD readings.

94. Answer: D

Answer: PPD containing 5 TU of tuberculin without controls.
The use of "control" testing is no longer recommended by the American Thoracic Society or the CDC for any patient routinely. Therefore, the use of controls should be discouraged. Even though she is severely immunocompromised, a standard PPD is still appropriate. **Never, ever** pick the 250 TU on a test. There is no reason to use it, so you can effectively mark out those answers when you see them listed on a test! The 2-step (or boosted) PPD has no place in routine practice; it is generally reserved for people who are repeatedly tested, such as health care workers.

Board Testing Point: Recognize that use of "controls" is no longer recommended for tuberculin skin testing.

95. Answer: D

Answer: PPD reading at 72 hours of 7 mm in an asthmatic patient on 5 mg/day of prednisone.
According to the guidelines, the cut-off is 10 mm for this patient. All of the other patients require treatment; generally, you would use INH for 9 months in each of these other patients. If this patient had been on 15 mg or more of daily prednisone, then they would have met the criteria for therapy.

Board Testing Point: Know how to interpret PPD results.

96. Answer: E

Answer: None needed unless clinical symptoms/problems develop.
He is a healthy person without evidence of liver disorder. If he had evidence during the initial evaluation to suggest a liver disorder, then you would draw baseline serum alanine aminotransferase (ALT) and bilirubin. Baseline testing is also indicated for patients with HIV infection treated with HAART, pregnant women, women in the immediate postpartum period (within 3 months of delivery), persons with a history of chronic liver disease (hepatitis B or C, alcoholic hepatitis, or cirrhosis), persons who use alcohol regularly, and persons at risk for chronic liver disease. Baseline testing is **no longer** absolutely indicated in older persons (> 35 years old), although some experts recommend that baseline and scheduled ALT testing be done in those older than 35 years. For patients with chronic conditions on medications that could cause problems, testing may be warranted. After baseline testing, individuals may be followed every 2–4 weeks depending on the severity of their clinical condition or if baseline laboratory is abnormal.

All patients regardless of age or health status require **clinical** monitoring! This includes educating patients about signs and symptoms that might indicate a problem with the medication. These include any of the following: unexplained anorexia, nausea, vomiting, dark urine, icterus, rash, persistent paresthesias of the hand and feet, persistent fatigue, weakness or fever lasting 3 or more days, abdominal tenderness (especially right upper quadrant discomfort), easy bruising or bleeding, and arthralgia. Clinical monitoring begins at the first visit and should be done monthly.

Board Testing Point: Recognize that screening laboratory is generally not recommended for most patients on INH therapy.

97. Answer: C

Answer: Ethambutol toxicity.
Ethambutol is generally not hepatotoxic, but will cause problems with visual acuity, particularly color perceptions. The other agents are not associated with this problem.

Board Testing Point: Recognize the toxicity associated with ethambutol.

98. Answer: D

Answer: Lumbar puncture.
She has cryptococcal lung disease, and there is a high risk of dissemination to the central nervous system with this organism. You aren't really going to have to differentiate, say, a *Histoplasma* from a *Cryptococcus*, but you will need to know the more common organisms that an immunocompromised person gets. A person with lymphoma, like this patient, is at increased risk for cryptococcal infection, *Coccidioides* infection, and *Aspergillus* infection. If we had said she was from the San Joaquin Valley—then it is a no-brainer, right? *Aspergillus*, remember, is branching. If they show you *Cryptococcus,* they will likely show it to you with the nice capsule that you remember from 2nd year medical school microbiology.

Board Testing Point: Recognize the need for lumbar puncture in an immunocompromised patient with possible cryptococcal lung disease.

99. Answer: C

Answer: Nasal continuous positive airway pressure (CPAP).
The continuous pressure "splints" the nasopharynx open at night. Unfortunately, it is uncomfortable for many patients. Sleeping supine and using hypnotics actually would worsen obstructive sleep apnea-hypopnea (OSAH). Sleeping under a fan would not have any effect. The type of television show shouldn't affect this either—although I know of no scientific study to prove this wrong.

Board Testing Point: Know appropriate therapy for obstructive sleep apnea-hypopnea.

100. Answer: E

Answer: Squamous cell carcinoma.
Squamous cell more commonly involves the central/hilar area with local extension, and is the most likely cancer to cavitate. Also, it is most commonly associated with hypercalcemia (large cell is next). Adenocarcinoma and large cell are usually peripheral. Bronchoalveolar carcinoma is just a subtype of adenocarcinoma. Squamous and small cell are usually central (remember the S-S sounds like Sentral). With small cell, cavitation **never** occurs. So if you put together central lesions, this leaves squamous and small cell; then put in cavitation and that leaves only squamous. Plus, for an added bonus, squamous is the one most commonly to have hypercalcemia.

Board Testing Point: Recognize clinical characteristics of lung cancers based on their location and associated clinical findings.

101. Answer: D

Answer: Small cell carcinoma.
Let's put this together. It is central, which means it is either Small Cell or Squamous Cell (Remember S-S-"Sentral"). Now you presume from the information that the patient has SIADH, which generally is associated with small cell. Therefore, put together central carcinoma with SIADH and you get small cell as the answer. Adenocarcinoma, large cell, and bronchoalveolar (a type of adenocarcinoma) are usually peripheral.

Board Testing Point: Recognize clinical characteristics of lung cancers based on their location and associated clinical findings.

102. Answer: E

Answer: After surgical resection, no further therapy is indicated.
She has a very localized lesion to the lung and a small tumor ≤ 3 cm. She does not have any nodal involvement and has no metastases. Also, she has a non-small cell type of cancer, so surgical resection should be sufficient. She does not need further therapy at this point, and studies have shown that adjuvant chemotherapy for this stage is actually deleterious. If her tumor was > 3 cm and she was Stage 1B (no nodes, no metastases), some trials have indicated that adjuvant chemotherapy may be useful and could be considered because of the size of the tumor.

Board Testing Point: Know appropriate therapy for lung cancer.

103. Answer: A

Answer: *Coxiella burnetii.*
In this case, the fact that he worked with animal placentas should make you think about *Coxiella burnetii.* Remember, if you see some type of animal "placenta" or birthing event, consider *Coxiella burnetii.* Recent literature reported outbreaks with **cats**—so be suspicious if Tabby is around delivering kittens and people are getting pneumonia. The other clue that this might be *Coxiella* is the marked hepatosplenomegaly. This is one of those "pneumonia with splenomegaly" organisms.

Board Testing Point: Recognize clinical features associated with *Coxiella burnetii* infection.

104. Answer: D

Answer: Systemic corticosteroids and itraconazole.
The key here is that she has Allergic Bronchopulmonary Aspergillosis (ABPA). The standard therapy used to be steroids alone; however, recent data have shown that adding itraconazole to the steroid therapy is beneficial. If you see something fungal that is branching, it is likely *Aspergillus*, especially if there is "right-angle" or 90-degree branching. Amphotericin IV or as a gargle is inappropriate in this instance, and fluconazole has limited activity against *Aspergillus*.

Board Testing Point: Know how to treat allergic bronchopulmonary aspergillosis.

105. Answer: A

Answer: Alveolar hypoventilation alone.
The differential diagnosis of arterial hypoxemia includes all of the choices plus decreased diffusion and high altitude (low FiO_2). While this patient is at risk for aspiration pneumonia, pulmonary edema, and other underlying pulmonary pathology, a quick calculation of the A-a gradient on room air reveals a normal A-a gradient. [150 – (50 + 72 / 0.8] = A-a gradient of 10. The A-a gradient is increased in all causes of hypoxemia except hypoventilation and high altitude. We were not given any information that this patient was found on the summit of a 10,000-foot mountain; therefore, alveolar hypoventilation due to the presumed narcotic injection is the physiological mechanism for hypoxemia in this patient.

Board Testing Point: Understand how to interpret arterial blood gases.

106. Answer: C

Answer: Transfuse 2 units packed red blood cells.
This patient is still only partially resuscitated with evidence for both hemorrhagic shock and the hyperdynamic phase of SIRS (systemic inflammatory response syndrome). Most important is the continued acidosis, which is predominantly a metabolic acidosis and presumably a lactic acidosis indicating inadequate tissue perfusion. The best way to continue the resuscitation is to improve oxygen delivery (DO_2) to the tissues and monitor the ABG and lactate level to assess improvement. Oxygen delivery is determined by cardiac output, hemoglobin, and oxygen **saturation**. In this case, the CO is already high, and the oxygen saturation with a PO_2 of 85 is at least 90%. Increasing the PO_2 will not provide much more hemoglobin saturation. Therefore, the best way to improve oxygen delivery is to increase the hemoglobin through additional packed red cell transfusions. Increasing the minute ventilation to compensate for the metabolic acidosis will only mask the problem. Dobutamine will reduce the systemic vascular resistance even more, resulting in further hypotension. Dopamine will increase the blood pressure and cause further tachycardia with no improvement in oxygen delivery to the tissues.

Board Testing Point: Recognize the need for blood transfusion in a patient with appropriate clinical evidence of volume depletion and shock.

107. Answer: E

Answer: Exercise challenge test.
With a normal cardiovascular and pulmonary exam, the most likely cause of the episodic dyspnea in this patient under 40 years of age is exercise-induced bronchospasm (EIB). Because this bronchospasm is episodic and a reversible airways obstruction, spirometry performed while the patient is asymptomatic may well be normal. An exercise challenge test is the most direct way to establish a diagnosis of EIB. This usually involves 6 to 8 minutes of ergometer or treadmill exercise, sufficient to raise the heart rate to 85 percent of the predicted maximum. A test is generally considered positive if the FEV_1 falls by 10 percent or more, although a fall of 15 percent is more diagnostic.

Alternatively, surrogate tests to assess bronchial hyperresponsiveness (e.g., cold air hyperventilation, methacholine or histamine inhalation challenge) may be performed in specialized laboratories, but do not always correlate with the presence of EIB. If the patient had rales on the exam and was older, the possibility of an interstitial lung disease would have to be entertained, and an HRCT of the chest would be indicated. Remember: 10% of patients with interstitial lung disease will have a normal chest x-ray at the time of presentation. If the patient gave a history of chest pain or syncope with exertion, and physical exam revealed a right parasternal heave and an accentuated P2, then the diagnosis of pulmonary hypertension by echocardiography would be warranted. If an upper airway obstruction was suggested by the history—or the patient was found to have stridor—a flow-volume loop would be a good screening test for upper airway obstruction. A normal ABG with a normal A-a gradient would make a diffusing capacity limitation unlikely.

Board Testing Point: Know how to diagnose exercise-induced bronchospasm.

108. Answer: E

Answer: No pulmonary function tests prior to surgery.
Pre-operative PFTs and blood gasses are recommended for patients with underlying lung disease who are to undergo operative procedures that are in proximity to the diaphragm. An FEV_1 less than 1 liter and arterial blood gases revealing hypoxemia and/or respiratory acidosis would place the patient at a higher risk for postoperative pulmonary complications (prolonged mechanical ventilation, pneumonia, atelectasis). This patient requires no further testing because his asthma is stable and the procedure is not in proximity to the diaphragm.

Board Testing Point: Know current guidelines for pulmonary function tests prior to surgery.

109. Answer: D

Answer: Inhaled corticosteroid plus long-acting beta-agonist.
This patient has asthma that would be characterized as moderate-persistent by the National Asthma Education and Prevention Program Guidelines. As such, she should be on daily medication with an inhaled corticosteroid and a long-acting inhaled beta agonist; alternatively, you could prescribe medium doses of an inhaled corticosteroid alone. The emphasis on utilizing antiinflammatory therapies (inhaled corticosteroids) was a major focus on the NAEPP guidelines for any asthma patient characterized as mild-persistent or greater. This was to overcome the over-reliance on symptomatic relief with beta2-agonist inhalers and the rising number of asthma deaths (most clutching their beta-agonist inhalers and on no steroids!). A beta2-agonist inhaler must be available for symptomatic relief with the understanding that more frequent use of the beta-agonist inhaler indicates a need for stepped-up antiinflammatory therapy (higher-dose inhaled steroids, PO prednisone). Sustained release theophylline may help with nocturnal symptoms but has no antiinflammatory action. Inhaled cromolyn alone can take weeks to start working and is best used in atopic asthma in children.

Board Testing Point: Recognize how to implement clinical guidelines for treatment of asthma.

110. Answer: A

Answer: Nasal oxygen, 1–2 L/min with follow-up ABG in 20 minutes. Increase oxygen flow based on the ABG to a PO_2 of 55–60 mmHg.

The treatment imperative is to provide this patient with supplemental oxygen to achieve a hemoglobin saturation of 88–90%. This is to prevent further hypoxemia, which can cause cardiac arrhythmias and acute cor pulmonale. Oxygen supplementation may result in worsening respiratory acidosis. (HINT: **not** through reduction in respiratory drive—COPD patients are just like the rest of us in that our chemiotaxic centers for the control of ventilation are CO_2 sensitive, not O_2 driven!) Worsening respiratory acidosis can be detected only by ABGs, not pulse oximetry. If providing supplemental FiO_2 to achieve an oxygen saturation of 88–90% results in severe respiratory acidosis, then positive pressure ventilation via non-invasive methods or conventional ventilation must be considered.

Board Testing Point: Recognize how to treat a severe COPD exacerbation.

111. Answer: D

Answer: Delayed (Type IV, cell mediated) skin test reaction to *Aspergillus fumigatus*.

All of the other choices are considered minor or major criteria for the diagnosis of ABPA, except that there is no Type IV, cell-mediated skin reaction. There are Type I and Type III (erythema and induration) skin test reactions. ABPA should be a consideration in any asthmatic who clinically worsens with repeated attacks despite adherence to therapy.

Board Testing Point: Recognize the clinical features associated with *Aspergillus fumigatus*.

112. Answer: D

Answer: Cryptogenic organizing pneumonia (COP).

While histologic confirmation is warranted, this is a classic presentation of COP. The flu-like illness that has not responded to antibiotics is a favorite of the ABIM. Histologic confirmation is needed because the patient will need a prolonged course (6–12 months) of corticosteroids and possible additional immunosuppressive agents. ABPA is unlikely because there is no prior history of asthma. Loeffler's is a self-limiting, benign eosinophilic pneumonia that is asymptomatic. IPF or other interstitial lung diseases are in the differential, but the time course is a little short and we have no occupational, environmental, or medication history. Hypersensitivity pneumonitis is not suggested by the history, and frequently the patient would appear more ill and have basilar rales on auscultation.

Board Testing Point: Recognize cryptogenic organizing pneumonia.

113. Answer: B

Answer: Echocardiogram.
Look for the young woman with exertional dyspnea, chest pain, and has physical exam findings consistent with right heart strain. The next step in the workup is an echocardiogram to document the existence of pulmonary hypertension and exclude significant mitral stenosis. After echocardiographic documentation of pulmonary hypertension, the workup would proceed in the absence of any discernible parenchymal lung disease to V/Q scan to look for thromboembolic disease. A pulmonary angiogram would be helpful in evaluating any perfusion defects seen on V/Q. The role of right heart catheterization is further down the road when you are considering vasodilator therapy in the patient with primary pulmonary hypertension.

We do not suspect cardiac ischemia. Pulmonary function tests (particularly diffusion capacity) are helpful in assessing severity in documented cases of pulmonary hypertension, but have little use in the initial workup of the patient unless you suspect secondary pulmonary hypertension from underlying COPD.

Board Testing Point: Recognize pulmonary hypertension and that echocardiogram is an appropriate diagnostic test.

114. Answer: A

Answer: Tuberculosis.
This effusion is clearly exudative, hemorrhagic, and with a lymphocytic predominance. There were no mesothelial cells noted. Tuberculosis pleuritis is common in elderly patients and should be a leading consideration in this case. Confirmation via fluid AFB stain and culture and/or pleural biopsy with culture should be performed. The absence of parenchymal or nodal disease leads us away from suspecting parapneumonic, lymphoma, or bronchogenic carcinoma. The negative pleural cytology rules out malignant mesothelioma.

Board Testing Point: Recognize the clinical manifestations of tuberculosis.

115. Answer: E

Answer: No testing or therapy.
This patient has acute histoplasmosis from the neighborhood barn-cleaning party. The neighborhood outbreak is not uncommon when there is land cleared or bulldozed. The key is that histoplasmosis is usually a self-limited disease for which we do not consider treatment unless there is evidence for progression to more disseminated disease. Some would consider treatment if symptoms persist more than 4 weeks, but before then treatment is not indicated by current guidelines. Treatment for mild disease that has persisted longer than 4 weeks would be with itraconazole, not amphotericin B, which is reserved for severe or disseminated disease. Accurate diagnosis relies on the history of exposure. Histoplasmin skin tests are useless, because many people will test positive after exposure without having the disease. Cultures are not very sensitive and may take weeks to grow. A positive culture from sputum or tissue is diagnostic, however. Serologic testing has variable sensitivity but would be the best test to diagnose her definitively; however, amphotericin B is not indicated.

Board Testing Point: Recognize that most patients with mild histoplasmosis do not require therapy.

116. Answer: D

Answer: Obtain prior chest x-rays for comparison.
When a lung lesion is first identified in a patient, it is imperative to determine whether the lesion is, in fact, new or old. If the lesion is old, you want to evaluate the stability of the lesion (no appreciable growth over 2 years.) Therefore, the first step is to obtain any old films. If there are no prior films, the next step is a high-resolution CT scan of the chest to evaluate the presence of disease. Or, if the old films are suspicious for growth, the CT scan is also indicated. Generally, in most cases your next step after looking at old plain films is to proceed with a high-resolution CT scan. If abnormalities are demonstrated, then bronchoscopy is indicated (if the lesion is amenable) to look for endobronchial involvement and rule out an infectious etiology for the lesion. If bronchoscopy is not helpful, there is some controversy as to whether it is best to perform transthoracic needle biopsy or just go to surgical removal of the lesion. The decision involves whether your patient would tolerate a thoracotomy and whether a non-diagnostic transthoracic needle biopsy (atypia, inflammatory Schmutz) would just mandate a thoracotomy anyway.

Board Testing Point: Know to always check for prior chest x-rays in a patient with an abnormality on current chest x-ray.

117. Answer: B

Answer: Order polysomnography with trial of nasal continuous positive airway pressure (CPAP).
The probability of this patient having serious obstructive sleep apnea is high. Therefore, a "split-study" polysomnography should be ordered such that the technician performing the study can analyze the results during the first part of the study and institute a trial of nasal CPAP if the preliminary result is unequivocally positive for serious obstructive sleep apnea (greater than 15 significant apnea/hypopnea events per hour). In this way, a patient can be started on nocturnal nasal CPAP as soon as possible. While weight loss, alcohol avoidance, and exercise are important instructions, it is unlikely that these measures alone will work in the short term in this patient. Uvulopalatopharyngoplasty is an alternative treatment for obstructive sleep apnea, but the results to date are inferior to CPAP. Theophylline and acetazolamide have not been shown in clinical trials to be beneficial.

Board Testing Point: Know the workup and therapy for obstructive sleep apnea-hypopnea.

118. Answer: B

Answer: Assist/control mode, Rate 12/min, Tidal Volume 700cc, Peak flow 80 L/min.
We all recognize that the hemodynamic demise in this patient was from dynamic hyperinflation and the creation of auto-PEEP. Just think of air trapping and breath "stacking." This patient's underlying problem is expiratory airflow obstruction. So what did the emergency department doctor do? In an effort to immediately reverse the acute hypercapnic respiratory failure, he hyperventilated the patient and provided a large tidal volume at a low peak flow rate. (Peak flow determines how fast the gas is delivered for each breath—a higher peak flow results in the breath being delivered quickly [short inspiratory time], allowing for a longer expiratory phase.) This patient could not possibly have had enough time to empty his lungs with each breath. Ultimately he builds up such a large pressure in his chest (auto-PEEP) that blood flow return is compromised and hypotension ensues. In removing the patient from mechanical ventilation, you allowed the trapped gas to be released and hemodynamic stability returned. While tempting to leave the patient on a T-bar without any positive pressure, I assure you that he will quickly tire and have a respiratory arrest.

Therefore, you return the patient to mechanical ventilation (assist/control mode is as good as any), with the understanding that you want a tidal volume of 5–10 mL/kg, a high peak flow rate, and a lower respiratory rate (8–14). Even without sophisticated monitoring, you should be able to see that you are not trapping air by auscultating the lungs through a few respiratory cycles and see that the patient has finished his expiration phase before the next breath by the ventilator is delivered. Recognize that this method of ventilating the patient may well not fully correct his respiratory acidosis. That's OK; a moderate amount of respiratory acidosis is well tolerated (permissive hypercapnia), so aim to get a pH > 7.20 as your initial goal and let the bronchodilators, steroids, etc., start to work.

Board Testing Point: Recognize the dynamics of auto-PEEP and how to alleviate the iatrogenic problem.

119. Answer: A

Answer: High cardiac output, low systemic vascular resistance, and low wedge pressure.
Utilizing a Swan-Ganz catheter to generate a hemodynamic profile of shock, such as in this case, is a reasonable question for the exam. They may even throw in more data such as pulmonary artery pressure, mixed venous oxygen saturation, and even left ventricular stroke volume to foul you up. Stick to the parameters above and you should be able to narrow down the answer sufficiently.

Remember: The hallmark of early, "warm" sepsis is a hyperdynamic heart (increased cardiac output) coupled with a **very low systemic vascular resistance**. Typically the patient in early septic shock is volume depleted and "third spacing" a considerable amount of the fluids given for resuscitation due to the low systemic vascular resistance. In all the other options listed, the systemic vascular resistance is high because it is the only thing holding the blood pressure together!

Volume depletion due to hypovolemic shock (whether hemorrhagic or intravascular) is characterized by a low wedge pressure, a reduced cardiac output, and a high SVR. Cardiogenic shock is defined by a low cardiac output, high-filling pressures (think CHF), and a high SVR. Obstructive shock is typified by a massive PE or a tension pneumothorax. There is reduced cardiac filling, reduced cardiac output, and a high SVR. In pericardial tamponade, the filling pressures will be normal as a reduced volume is acted on by a decreased compliance of the ventricular wall.

Board Testing Point: Know how to use Swan-Ganz catheter results to determine the likely etiology of shock.

120. Answer: C

Answer: Order a quantitative ventilation scan.
The only cure for lung cancer is a surgical resection. As such, we strive to make any patient a surgical candidate. This patient's pre-op PFTs show an FEV_1 less than 2.0 liters—the traditional cutoff for surgical candidates. Smoking cessation, inhaled steroids, and further intervention from a pulmonologist may improve his FEV_1, but at the risk of delaying the curative procedure. Therefore, since there are asymmetrical bullae on the CT scan, it is likely that the ventilation scan will show less ventilation to the right lung, and a quantitative assessment would allow even a right pneumonectomy.

Board Testing Point: Know how to manage a patient who is due for lung resection and has a low FEV_1.

121. Answer: B

Answer: Order an ECG and echocardiogram to evaluate for cor pulmonale.
For insurance to cover this man's home oxygen, you would need to demonstrate evidence of cor pulmonale in addition to his blood gas results. His Hct does not qualify him on the basis of erythrocytosis.

These are the current indications for continuous long-term oxygen therapy for patients with chronic lung disease:

1) Resting $P_aO_2 \leq 55$ mmHg, **or**
2) O_2 saturation $\leq 88\%$, **or**
3) $P_aO_2 \leq 59$ mmHg (O_2 sat $\leq 89\%$) with evidence of cor pulmonale

Evidence of cor pulmonale in these considerations is:

- Clinical evidence of right heart failure
- Pulmonale on ECG (p wave height > 2.5 mm in II, III, and AVF
- Hct > 5.6 (due to polycythemia from chroinic hypoxia 2° cor pulmonale)

Medicare guidelines require you to bring him back between 61 and 90 days and retest him. Note that the use of supplemental oxygen does **not** depress the respiratory drive and cause an elevated CO_2. This is due to several factors, including an easing of pulmonary vasoconstriction, which leads to perfusion of previously underperfused spaces and possibly due to ventilation of previous dead space.

Board Testing Point: Know the guidelines for continuous long-term oxygen therapy for patients with chronic lung disease.

122. Answer: B

Answer: Bilateral peripheral infiltrates.
This presentation of a 40-year-old woman with a history of fever, night sweats, asthma exacerbation, and new eosinophilia is classic for chronic eosinophilic pneumonia. The CXR is classically referred to as the "photographic negative" of pulmonary edema. ABPA would be suggested by a history of coughing brownish sputum and the subsequent mucous plugging that can lead to segmental atelectasis on chest x-ray. There is always a possibility of pulmonary tuberculosis (right upper lobe cavity), but the eosinophilia would not be a hallmark.

Board Testing Point: Recognize the clinical and radiographic findings of chronic eosinophilic pneumonia.

123. Answer: D

Answer: High-resolution CT of the chest.
Nearly 10% of patients presenting with interstitial lung disease will have a normal CXR. High-resolution chest CT is the test of choice to evaluate for the presence of an interstitial lung disease. HRCT will be helpful diagnostically in assessing the distribution of the disease as well as providing guidance for a possible lung biopsy. In addition, HRCT may provide a clue to the staging of the disease (ground-glass appearing airspace disease suggests an active cellular component vs. burnt out fibrosis). This case is a little different from a similar case you saw elsewhere; here, the CXR is normal and thus you would want more information/data (HRCT) before proceeding directly to bronchoalveolar lavage and/or transbronchial biopsy.

Full PFTs would merely provide confirmation of what you already suspect: This patient has an interstitial lung disease with probably restricted lung volumes and a reduced diffusing capacity. Flexible bronchoscopy with transbronchial biopsy could be entertained if we felt a strong suspicion for sarcoid or an infectious etiology. The yield on transbronchial biopsy is very good for these etiologies. However, in order to provide an adequate tissue sample for examination in most ILDs, an open lung biopsy (traditional or thoracoscopic) is required—but again, we would wait on the HRCT first.

Board Testing Point: Evaluate a patient with possible interstitial lung disease but who has a normal CXR.

124. Answer: B

Answer: Non-caseating granulomatous inflammatory changes.
She has multi-organ involvement to suggest the diagnosis of sarcoidosis. The initial lesions on her legs were probably those of erythema nodosum. A biopsy would have found a probable panniculitis at that time. Hypercalcemia, facial nerve palsy, and cutaneous involvement are, again, typical. ACE levels may be elevated, but not always. A chest x-ray would probably be appropriate as part of her workup. Non-caseating granulomas are charactertistic of sarcoidosis.

Board Testing Point: Recognize the histologic findings in a skin biopsy associated with sarcoidosis.

125. Answer: D

Answer: Start azithromycin at 250 mg PO daily.
This patient has high-risk COPD based on the severity of his FEV_1 predicted and the number of exacerbations per year. He has already been treated as per guidelines with antiinflammatories and long-acting bronchodilators. He has quit smoking, receives indicated vaccinations, has engaged in pulmonary rehabilitation, and has been assessed for oxygen treatment.

Azithromycin has been evaluated in patients with severe COPD with frequent exacerbations. When given at a dose of 250 mg PO daily, it was associated with reductions in exacerbation and increased the time to first exacerbation. It would be a reasonable treatment option for this patient assuming relative contraindications do not exist. Caution must be used given the potential of adverse reactions related to hearing impairment and QT prolongation.

Based on his testing, neither increasing his oxygen level nor initiating non-invasive ventilation in the absence of hypercarbia will prove beneficial. Chronic systemic steroids are associated with many adverse effects and have been associated with increased morbidity and mortality and thus are not recommended. Lung transplantation could be considered, although, in the setting of COPD, is a complex algorithm. There are many variables to consider, but these include an $FEV_1 < 25\%$ predicted, evidence of hypercarbia, and resting hypoxemia. This patient does not meet those criteria.

Board Testing Point: Know indications for azithromycin in a patient with severe COPD with frequent exacerbations.

126. Answer: D

Answer: Obtain a polysomnography exam.
This patient has clinical evidence to suggest pulmonary hypertension that is supported by the findings of the echocardiogram. This is further classified by the World Health Organization as:

Group I: Includes disorders in which the pulmonary hypertension is associated with abnormalities in the small branches of the pulmonary artery, the arterioles. Several types of pulmonary hypertension are in Group I, including idiopathic pulmonary hypertension, and pulmonary hypertension due to several types of infection, connective tissue disorders, and some types of congenital heart disease.

Group II: This group includes pulmonary hypertension caused by left-sided heart disease.

Group III: This group includes pulmonary hypertension due to hypoxemia, including chronic lung disease and obstructive sleep apnea.

Group IV: This group includes pulmonary hypertension due to pulmonary thromboembolic disease.

Group V: This group includes pulmonary hypertension due to other miscellaneous causes that do not fit into the other four categories.

The evaluation of a patient with signs and symptoms associated with pulmonary hypertension starts with consideration of diagnosis that may explain the symptoms. Echocardiogram is the screening test of choice to evaluate for pulmonary hypertension since it is non-invasive and has reasonable sensitivity. If pulmonary hypertension is suggested by the echocardiogram findings, then causes of secondary types of PAH (WHO Groups II–V) should be evaluated.

For this patient, consideration for obstructive sleep apnea must be taken, given his endorsement of snoring, restless sleep, and elevated BMI.

Given the history of recent long travel prior to symptoms, it is reasonable to consider venous thromboembolic disease. However, the pre-test probability is low, the disease has chronicity, and the patient is clinically stable. Initiation of anti-coagulation with low molecular weight heparin would not be appropriate without further diagnostic information to confirm the diagnosis.

If the evaluation of secondary causes of pulmonary hypertension does not provide a good explanation for the elevated pressures, then proceeding with a pulmonary artery catheterization at that time would be an appropriate step. Initiation of pulmonary vasodilators, such as sildenafil or epoprostenol, is indicated for WHO Group I Pulmonary arterial hypertension. They should not be initiated until secondary causes of pulmonary hypertension are excluded and elevated PA pressures are documented by pulmonary artery catheterization.

Board Testing Point: Know the workup of pulmonary hypertension.

127. Answer: A

Answer: Perform tube thoracostomy.

This patient has evidence of an empyema. He has developed a large left-sided unilateral effusion in the setting of recent pneumonia. This is associated with the development of sepsis. The pleural fluid studies are consistent with an empyema based on the visual evidence of pus. A positive Gram stain also would be indicative of an empyema, but the absence of this does not exclude the diagnosis. Additionally, the following results are indicative of an empyema or a complicated para pneumonic effusion:

- pH < 7.2
- Glucose < 60
- LDH > 1,000
- WBC > 50,000

An empyema will require drainage to prevent further complications; hence, tube thoracostomy is the best answer. Repeat thoracentesis is unlikely to allow complete drainage and would not be an appropriate option. Treatment with antibiotics alone would be reasonable to consider in a patient with a simple parapneumonic effusion, but not for empyema. There is no other evidence to suggest that this effusion is related to pulmonary edema or congestive heart failure. Although CHF is the most common reason for effusions, they are unilateral to the left < 10% of the time and would be associated with a transudative effusion. Thus, furosemide would not be indicated.

Board Testing Point: Recognize an empyema and know the treatment.

128. Answer: E

Answer: Discharge home on leuofloxacin.

The patient has community-acquired pneumonia (CAP). Severity of illness is the most critical factor in making the determination for admission. The pneumonia severity index (PSI) is a 20-item calculation that is pretty complicated. The CURB-65 is a derivative test that is almost as accurate and much simpler! CURB-65 prognostic variables: **C**onfusion, **U**rea (BUN > 20 mg/dL), **R**espiratory rate ≥ 30 breaths/minute, **B**lood pressure (systolic < 90 mmHg or diastolic ≤ 60 mmHg), and age ≥ **65** years. 0–1 = low-risk; 2 = mod-risk; 3–5 = high-risk. This patient scores 0 out of 5, so he can be managed as an outpatient.

Streptococcus pneumoniae is the most common bacterial cause of CAP. Influenza is the most common viral cause. Other common bacterial causes are *Mycoplasma pneumonia* and *Legionella*.

For CAP patients with no comorbidities, treat as an outpatient with either oral azithromycin or doxycycline. However, this patient has COPD, and the presence of significant comorbidities (COPD, liver or renal disease, cancer, diabetes, chronic heart disease, alcoholism, asplenia, or immunosuppression), and/or use of antibiotics within the prior 3 months, increases the risk of infection with drug-resistant *S. pneumoniae* (DRSP).

Therefore, in this case, treat the patient with either azithromycin or doxycycline **plus** a beta lactam that has activity against DRSP (amox-clavulanic, cefpodoxime, or cefuroxime). Alternatively, treat with a respiratory fluoroquinolone (levofloxacin, gemifloxacin, or moxifloxacin).

Patients with CAP should be appropriately vaccinated for influenza and pneumococcal infection. This patient's COPD qualifies him for pneumococcal immunization.

Board Testing Point: Know the management of CAP in an outpatient with risk factor for DRSP.

129. Answer: A

Answer: Start vancomycin, plus a respiratory fluoroquinolone.
The patient described above appears to have been initially admitted with a viral pneumonia related to influenza A infection. The systemic symptoms, chest radiograph picture, and positive influenza culture support this as the initial diagnosis.

Initial treatment with oseltamivir at 75 mg PO bid is appropriate and indicated for those hospitalized with influenza, patients with lower respiratory tract infection, and those with age > 65. Doubling the dose to 150 mg PO bid has been advocated for those with severe critical illness and those that may be immunosuppressed, although efficacy data are unclear. Oseltamivir has been demonstrated to shorten the duration of influenza symptoms and to reduce the duration of viral shedding. Some studies have also shown that oseltamivir reduces illness severity and complication rates.

The patient in this scenario certainly decompensated during the hospitalization with much higher fevers and new chest radiographic appearance. This is very concerning for new bacterial infection superimposed on viral influenza. The most common pathogens responsible for secondary bacterial complications are *Streptococcus pneumoniae*, *Streptococcus pyogenes*, and *Staphylococcus aureus*. For this reason, empiric coverage with vancomycin plus a respiratory fluoroquinolone is the best option.

Board Testing Point: Know of the increased tendency of bacterial lung infections due to a viral influenza. Know the empiric treatment for bacterial pneumonia.

130. Answer: C

Answer: This patient should start annual low-dose CT screening for lung cancer.
Lung cancer is the leading cause of cancer-related death among men and women with increasing rates of cancer-related deaths worldwide. The great majority, up to 75%, of lung cancer presents at an advanced stage that is not amenable to cure. For this reason, there has been substantial evaluation regarding methods for lung screening.

Despite multiple studies, screening with chest radiographs, sputum cytology, or both of those modalities combined, have not demonstrated any benefit in terms of mortality from lung cancer.

In contrast, screening for lung cancer with low-dose CT has been shown to be effective. Specifically, the NLST, which was a trial of CT screening in patients at high risk, demonstrated a reduction in lung cancer mortality by nearly 20%. As a result of this large trial, most expert groups have now recommended screening for lung cancer. Most recently, the U.S. Preventive Services Task Force (USPSTF) revised its guidelines in 2013 based on this study and a larger meta-analysis. Those current recommendations are for annual low-dose CT scan for:

- High-risk adults 55 to 80 years old
- 30 pack-year smoking history and current smoker, or quit within the past 15 years
- Discontinuation of screening once the individual has not smoked for 15 years, or has a limited life expectancy

Board Testing Point: Know which at-risk groups should be screened for lung cancer—and best test for screening.

131. Answer: D

Answer: Skin testing for reactivity to *Aspergillus fumigatus*.
This scenario represents a classic example of allergic bronchopulmonary aspergillosis (ABPA). This is a recurrent hypersensitivity reaction in response to bronchial colonization by *Aspergillus*, and is a common cause of poorly controlled asthma. Bronchial obstruction by mucus and chronic inflammation can lead to bronchiectasis and lung fibrosis with irreversible loss of lung function. Symptoms include productive cough, frequent bronchitis or asthma exacerbations, and dyspnea and wheezing. Patients universally have a history of asthma and the diagnosis is often delayed as patients are treated for asthma and frequently improve when placed on systemic steroids. Diagnostic features include:

- Immediate reactivity on skin prick with *Aspergillus* antigens
- Precipitating serum antibodies to *A. fumigatus*
- Serum total IgE concentration > 1,000 ng/mL
- Peripheral blood eosinophilia > 500/mm^3
- Lung opacities on chest x-ray or chest HRCT
- Central bronchiectasis present on chest CT
- Elevated specific serum IgE and IgG to *A. fumigatus*

A skin test is the best first test, because it is 100% sensitive (i.e., a negative test rules out the condition). A serum IgE < 1,000 or negative precipitating antibodies also rule out ABPA with high confidence.

Testing for cystic fibrosis and HIV are part of a thorough workup for unexplained bronchiectasis, but skin testing for *Aspergillus* reactivity should come first. Omalizumab is indicated for people with severe persistent asthma with positive allergy skin testing and IgE levels ~ 75 to 1,750 ng/mL. It has not been studied extensively in the setting of ABPA.

Board Testing Point: Recognize ABPA and the best initial test for ruling it out.

132. Answer: B

Answer: 3 months.
According to the ACCP guidelines, pulmonary embolism or other VTE with a clear provoking factor should be treated with warfarin for 3 months. In the setting when a provoking factor is present, testing for thrombophilia is not recommended. Additionally, the evidence is sparse and unclear regarding the efficacy of thrombophilia screening after unprovoked VTE. Those patients with common thrombophilic conditions such as heterozygosity for factor V Leiden or prothrombin mutation are at a slightly increased risk for recurrent VTE. However, this does not mean that lifelong anticoagulation is warranted when a provoking factor is present.

In the case of unprovoked VTE, testing for recognized hypercoagulable states is not necessarily recommended either. Patients with a first episode of acute unprovoked VTE should receive anticoagulant therapy for 3 months and then be reassessed. Continued anticoagulation is in part determined by the bleeding risk of the patient because the recurrence rate can be as high as 25% over the next 5 years. Those who have a low-to-moderate risk of bleeding may benefit from the continuation of therapy indefinitely. Conversely, those who have a high risk of bleeding may benefit from the discontinuation of therapy after 3 months. This decision should be individualized.

In regard to the timing of thrombophilia testing, it is important to understand how anticoagulation affects certain labs. Treatment will invalidate the results for antithrombin III, protein C and S, and lupus anticoagulants; thus, these should not be assessed for at least 2 weeks after stopping anticoagulation. Anticoagulation does not affect the results for *Factor V Leiden*, hyperhomocysteinemia, and the cardiolipin and B2-glycoprotein antibody tests.

Board Testing Point: Know the duration of warfarin treatment when given for VTE with a clear provoking factor.

133. Answer: C

Answer: Continue to monitor.
This patient has a submassive pulmonary embolism (PE) which is characterized by signs of RV dysfunction (elevated neck veins) but without severe hypotension (i.e., SBP > 90). The management for submassive pulmonary embolism remains somewhat controversial. The use of t-PA and other thrombolytics has been shown to accelerate clot lysis and provide short-lived hemodynamic benefits. It also may lessen the risk of requiring escalation of therapy such as t-PA later. The impact on longer-term pulmonary hypertension is still not clear. There is, however, an increased risk of major bleeding, and no studies have clearly demonstrated a mortality reduction or reduced rates of recurrence.

This patient has remained relatively stable, and an echocardiogram has not been performed, which makes the demonstration of right ventricular dysfunction not yet clear. For this reason, continued monitoring while on heparin is the next best step. Additionally, her clinical status does not warrant the need for intubation.

The ACCP guidelines support the use of thrombolytics in patients with massive pulmonary embolus (associated with shock, SBP < 90) although the grade of evidence is considered weak. Additionally, they recommend that most patients without hypotension should not be treated with thrombolytics. They do, however, offer consideration for those with significant RV enlargement by CTA or echocardiogram, as well as those who become increasingly unstable. The risk of bleeding must also be factored into any decision, as severe bleeding may occur in up to 20% of recipients of thrombolytics, with up to 3% suffering intracranial hemorrhage.

Surgical thrombectomy should be considered only in those with massive pulmonary embolus in which t-PA or catheter-directed thrombolysis has not been effective. It carries a very high morbidity and mortality rate and has not been well studied. The practice of placing an IVC filter in those with a large deep venous thrombosis is not supported by evidence. It should be considered only in those for whom anticoagulation is not feasible or those deemed to be at significant cardiovascular risk if residual clot does migrate to the pulmonary artery. The presence of a lower extremity DVT should be confirmed prior to an IVC filter.

Board Testing Point: Know when to treat pulmonary emboli with thrombolytics.

CARDIOLOGY

134. Answer: D

Answer: Decrease in systolic BP > 15 mmHg.
Other things that should make you stop the test quickly are: ST-segment depression greater than 2 mm; development of ventricular tachycardias; development of severe chest pain, shortness of breath, or lightheadedness. His target heart rate is ~ 148 bpm because that represents 85% of his maximum predicted heart rate of 175 bpm (220-age). Remember that a positive test is indicated by finding ST depression of > 1 mm at the J+80 millisecond point in 2 contiguous leads. His prior probability of heart disease is very high based on his symptoms and family history, so a positive test in this patient is likely a true positive.

Board Testing Point: Know the reasons to stop a treadmill stress test emergently.

135. Answer: C

Answer: Insertion of a permanent cardiac pacemaker.
What the ECG is describing is the sudden failure of atrial ventricular conduction without a preceding change in the PR interval. The patient has Mobitz type 2, 2nd degree AV block. This is **bad** and usually means significant disease of the conducting system. It is also an unstable thing to have and frequently will progress to complete heart block. Additionally, he is severely symptomatic. Therefore, the only correct solution is to put in a permanent pacemaker in anticipation that he will continue to have worsening of his conduction abnormalities.

Board Testing Point: Recognize the clinical features of Mobitz type 2, 2nd degree AV block, and know that the likely therapy in a symptomatic patient will require permanent pacemaker placement.

136. Answer: C

Answer: Decrease of the murmur with handgrip.
His echocardiogram showing evidence of a disproportionately thickened ventricular septum and systolic anterior motion of the mitral valve strongly suggests hypertrophic cardiomyopathy, also known as idiopathic hypertrophic subaortic stenosis (IHSS). The harsh systolic murmur that he has should not radiate to the carotids with this condition. Additionally, the murmur will decrease when he applies a handgrip; this handgrip isometric exercise will increase systolic and diastolic blood pressure and, hence, increase afterload. This increase in afterload will decrease the murmur from HOCM. The carotid upstroke is brisk and frequently is bifid. His congestive failure is likely occurring because of the reduced ventricular compliance despite **normal** left ventricular systolic function. Mitral regurgitation is much more likely than mitral stenosis.

Board Testing Point: Know the clinical features of hypertrophic cardiomyopathy.

137. Answer: C

Answer: Diffuse T-wave inversion with ST-segment elevation.
Many of you probably went for the "no rub" answer. However, remember that a rub is actually not that common. So if we read the question as, "Which of the following findings **can** occur in acute pericarditis?" then the finding of "**no rub**" is certainly a possibility. **Now**, if the rub is there, it is diagnostic; if not, then it really doesn't help you rule out the diagnosis. With a pericarditis, you would expect to see frequent atrial premature beats. Also, PR-segment depression, especially in Lead II, would help you here. CPKs frequently will rise with pericarditis and in fact can be 2–3 times normal; but they are **transiently** elevated. The finding of diffuse T-wave inversion with ST-segment elevation more likely means the poor guy had an MI, not pericarditis. These ECG findings would **least** support the diagnosis of acute pericarditis.

Board Testing Point: Recognize the clinical findings of acute pericarditis.

138. Answer: A

Answer: Bicuspid aortic valve.
70% of people with coarctation will also have a bicuspid aortic valve. Usually, signs such as murmurs don't occur until later in life in the mid-30s. None of the other conditions is commonly associated with coarctation. She does have Turner syndrome. Note also that aneurysms of the circle of Willis occur with coarctation.

Board Testing Point: Recognize the association of coarctation with bicuspid aortic valve.

139. Answer: C

Answer: Add an ACE inhibitor.
Clinical presentation is consistent with heart failure. Considering presence of S_3 gallop, he likely has HF with reduced EF. He needs appropriate medical therapy and echocardiogram (the most useful diagnostic test in the evaluation of patients with heart failure). Adding the ACE inhibitor will increase cardiac output and decrease LV filling pressure due to the vasodilatory effect. ACE inhibitors block formation of angiotensin II, causing an increase in renin (from decreased negative feedback). They have been shown to reduce morbidity and mortality in patients with systolic HF. Increasing the digoxin dose would not be a good idea based on his current digoxin level (dose should actually be reduced to achieve serum levels between 0.5 and 1.0). There is no need to go to a loop diuretic at this point because the hydrochlorothiazide is working well. A calcium channel blocker would not be effective and could be harmful due to a possible negative inotropic effect. Beta-blocker is not given as an option but would obviously be necessary in the future, particularly if echocardiogram confirms reduced LV EF; beta-blockers are generally added once a patient is euvolemic.

Board Testing Point: Know that an ACE inhibitor is the 1st drug for treatment of CHF and should be part of any management plan for CHF.

140. Answer: C

Answer: Decrease the propranolol dose.
Be aware that some patients may have an increased sensitivity to the effects of beta-blockers. The easiest thing is to decrease the dosing interval to twice a day and see if that works. The other tests are not indicated. Remember, he is asymptomatic, so insertion of a temporary pacemaker is not indicated at this point.

Board Testing Point: Board Testing Point: Know that certain patients may have an increased sensitivity to beta-blockers.

141. Answer: B

Answer: Initial placement of the orthodontic bands.
According to the ACC/AHA 2008 Guideline Update on Valvular Heart Disease: Focused Update on Infective Endocarditis, prophylaxis prior to dental procedures is now indicated only for patients with specific highest-risk-for-IE cardiac conditions:

- Prosthetic valves (bioprosthetic or mechanical)
- Previous episode of endocarditis
- Congenital heart disease (CHD)
    - Unrepaired cyanotic CHD
    - Repaired CHD within 6 months of procedure
    - Repaired CHD with residual defects
- Cardiac transplant patients with valve lesions

Prophylaxis is no longer indicated for bicuspid aortic valve, any ASD or VSD (unless unrepaired and cyanotic, or repaired with residual defect), native valvular stenosis or regurgitation, mitral valve prolapse (with or without murmur), coronary artery bypass graft (CABG), or HCM (unless repair occurs within 6 months of procedure).

Regarding dental procedures in these patients with highest-risk-for-IE conditions, antibiotic prophylaxis is given only for dental procedures that involve manipulation of gingival tissue or the periapical region of teeth or perforation of the oral mucosa. This includes the initial placement of orthodontics bands but not the subsequent periodic adjustments. Oral suture removal does not require antibiotic prophylaxis.

Board Testing Point: Only area patients with the highest risk for of adverse outcomes with IE are prophylaxed for specific dental procedures—those that have significant gum manipulation or bleeding require antibiotic prophylaxis.

142. Answer: E

Answer: None of the choices is correct.
He is at **high** risk because of his prosthetic valve. Other high-risk conditions include previous endocarditis and those with surgically constructed systemic pulmonary shunts or conduits. However, genitourinary procedures do not have a significant risk of bacteremia, and as such, prophylaxis is no longer recommended for genitourinary or gastrointestinal procedures.

Board Testing Point: Know that the latest guidelines do not recommend antibiotic prophylaxis for any genitourinary or gastrointestinal procedure, even in patients with prosthetic cardiac valves.

143. Answer: B

Answer: Atenolol.
A patient like this, with both hypertension and ischemic heart disease, really does warrant the use of a beta-adrenolytic agent so that the "cardio-protective" properties of this drug family may be employed. In a patient with both obstructive pulmonary disease and peripheral vascular disease with claudication, this would be the perfect scenario for the preferential use of the selective agent such as atenolol (or metoprolol, etc.). Use of propranolol in this setting would likely add a bronchospastic component such that the patient's COPD could worsen. ACE inhibitors are not considered a usual treatment for angina pectoris alone. To date, there are conflicting data regarding a possible benefit in reducing exercise-induced angina. Obviously, ACE inhibitors are becoming 1st line for therapy of hypertension, particularly in diabetic patients. Other agents proven useful in management of angina pectoris include nitrates and calcium channel blockers.

Board Testing Point: Recognize that beta-blockers are considered the drug of choice for treatment of angina pectoris.

144. Answer: A

Answer: A calcium antagonist given intravenously (IV) cannot be selected safely as the initial treatment.
While absolute statements are seldom possible in medicine, one in which you may be confident is the following: "Calcium antagonism is **never** the treatment for a patient with wide complex tachycardia in the emergency setting."

If the diagnosis were actually traditional ventricular tachycardia, the calcium antagonist would have no primary efficacy and would simply add the adverse effect of negative inotropicity. If the diagnosis were antidromic conduction of a supraventricular tachycardia in the setting of pre-excitation physiology, the calcium antagonist would retard conduction at the atrioventricular (AV) junction and thereby enhance anomalous antegrade conduction.

The majority of patients who present with ventricular tachycardia have underlying structural heart disease. However, there has been increasing appreciation of the existence of multiple forms of idiopathic ventricular tachycardia with distinct features and unique mechanisms. The most common form of idiopathic ventricular tachycardia originates from the right ventricular outflow tract, which is characterized by sensitivity to adenosine, and appears to be due to cyclic AMP-mediated triggered activity. Other forms of idiopathic ventricular tachycardia include intrafascicular left ventricular tachycardia due to reentry, which is sensitive to verapamil, and automatic, propranolol-sensitive ventricular tachycardia. Although the mechanism of verapamil-sensitive idiopathic left ventricular tachycardia (ILVT) is usually reentry, the actual reentrant circuit is not clearly understood. This latter entity would be the sole exception to the general rule stated above, one that would not apply directly to the acute scenario as described.

Board Testing Point: Understand that calcium channel blockers should never be the initial therapy for wide complex tachycardia in an emergent setting.

145. Answer: D

Answer: Right coronary artery (RCA).
This is the classic picture of inferior myocardial infarction and should correlate with occlusion of a right coronary artery.

Board Testing Point: Determine which coronary artery is involved based on clinical and ECG clues.

146. Answer: B

Answer: WPW with orthodromic tachycardia (AVRT).
The key to the correct diagnosis here is the noting of the QP interval (> 100 msec). In AVNRT, the P wave is hidden in the QRS complex. These are the patients with congenital dual AV pathways whose reentry loop is restricted to the area surrounding the AV node. In the patient with AVRT, the normal impulse during tachycardia will travel antegradely down the normal conduction pathway and then will use the Kent pathway for the retrograde limb of the reentry loop. What this means, however, is that there is a measurably longer distance and greater time needed for the advancing impulse to return to atrial myocardium in order to excite a P wave, the latter then being delayed and appearing "down the page" in the ensuing ST segment. Wenckebach (1st degree AV block with Mobitz 1 progression) would not explain tachycardia; WPW with antidromic tachycardia should be a **wide** complex tachycardia; and multifocal atrial tachycardia should be irregular. Some authors place the diagnostic threshold of the QP interval at shorter levels (e.g., 70 msec).

Board Testing Point: Recognize the ECG findings of WPW.

147. Answer: C

Answer: Enhanced automaticity.
Although not seen on a daily basis, the phenomenon of non-paroxysmal junctional tachycardia is exceedingly important both from a practical clinical point of view and a conceptual example. Arguably, this is the very best example of "enhanced automaticity," the junctional tissues having been accelerated nonspecifically by 1 or more of several factors such as the following:

1) Digitalis excess
2) Hypokalemia
3) Post-infarction state
4) Post-operative state
5) Post-prandial hypoglycemia
6) Other

Magnesium sulfate may have a role in treatment, although the usual focus is the correction of the spectrum of reversible contributors operative in the specific patient. The rate range of 70–130/min is very important, particularly given the overlap with the normal range for the resting sinoatrial node. By way of review, the junctional rhythms are:

##	Name	Rate Range	Significance
1	Junctional escape ("idionodal rhythm")	0–60/min	Default pacemaker
2	Non-paroxysmal junctional tachycardia (NPJT)	70–130/min	As above; never "normal" or "chronic"
3	Paroxysmal junctional tachycardia (PJT)	150–250/min	Rare, rapid, perhaps "incessant"

Board Testing Point: Understand the concept of enhanced automaticity.

148. Answer: C

Answer: Insert a long, large-bore needle into her left chest toward her cardiac apex.
This poor woman has had severe chest trauma. Her physical neck veins are consistent with acute tamponade, certainly from a traumatic hemopericardium. A tension pneumothorax would produce distended pulseless neck veins and absent breath sounds on 1 side. Rotating tourniquets was an old therapy for heart failure, which she could have conceivably had from coronary artery trauma and myocardial infarction, but the treatment would not have been sufficient.

Board Testing Point: Recognize the clinical features of cardiac tamponade and understand the emergent treatment.

149. Answer: A

Answer: Aortic regurgitation.
Aortic regurgitation tolerates exercise well because exercise does 2 good things: 1) dilates the peripheral vasculature, allowing more blood to move forward, and 2) produces tachycardia, which shortens the time for regurgitation during diastole. Exercise is contraindicated in aortic stenosis, hypertrophic cardiomyopathy, and in patients with Eisenmenger syndrome. Exercise is not dangerous in patients with mitral stenosis, but it is not well tolerated.

Board Testing Point: Recognize that aortic regurgitation usually will tolerate exercise well.

150. Answer: B

Answer: RV infarction with secondary failure; administer normal saline.
In this setting of a recent acute inferior MI and new recurrence of severe chest pain, you must be worried about RV infarction with secondary failure. The RV has decompensated and is unable to fill the left side. Initial treatment is to give fluids. Think of this in a hypotensive patient with inferior MI! The decompensated RV is dependent upon preload to maintain cardiac output; do NOT give these patients nitrates that will decrease preload. With pericardial tamponade, you would get equal diastolic pressures in all 4 chambers. In addition, the question might give hints in the physical exam such as distended neck veins and soft heart sounds.

For biventricular failure, you would expect low cardiac output, high PCWP, and high RA pressure. Treatment listed is correct.

With mitral stenosis with secondary RV failure, you would see elevated RA pressure, elevated PA press, and elevated PCWP.

In pulmonary hypertension, you would see that the RA pressure is elevated and the PA diastolic pressure is markedly higher than the PCWP. The PA pressures in this example are not markedly elevated.

Board Testing Point: Recognize the possible complications after a myocardial infarction.

---

151. Answer: D

Answer: Atrial fibrillation.
This patient had acute onset of symptoms. As it turns out, his aunt and uncle had protein C deficiency. And guess what? So does this guy. His atrial fibrillation resulted from a big pulmonary embolism. Note the baseline wandering representing the atrial fibrillation waves and fast, irregular ventricular response.

Board Testing Point: Recognize the ECG appearance of atrial fibrillation.

---

152. Answer: E

Answer: Amiodarone.
The most appropriate management of cardiac arrest induced by ventricular tachycardia (which is what the rhythm strip shows) is administering an initial 200-joule defibrillation. Additional shocks at higher energies, up to a maximum of 360 joules, should be attempted if the initial shock is ineffective in reverting the ventricular tachycardia. Current ACLS guidelines support the use of amiodarone as adjunctive therapy in patients refractory to cardioversion. If amiodarone is not available, lidocaine is an alternative. Remember, in patients with unstable arrhythmias (e.g., chest pain, SOB, hypotension, mental status changes), immediate cardioversion is most appropriate.

Board Testing Point: Know the ACLS protocol for pulseless V-tach.

---

153. Answer: A

Answer: Right heart failure.
Ankle edema does not equal heart failure! Look at her physical examination: She has no jugular venous distention—it is very, very unlikely for her to have heart failure with normal jugular pressures. All of the other items listed should be considered before you even think about right heart failure. Also remember that calcium channel blockers (e.g., amlodipine, nifedipine, diltiazem) used for treating HTN can also cause lower extremity edema by blunting postural cutaneous vasoconstriction.

Board Testing Point: Be able to list a differential diagnosis for peripheral leg edema in a patient without signs of right heart failure.

---

154. Answer: B

Answer: Parenteral penicillin and aspirin.
This patient has acute rheumatic fever. Remember: He needs 2 of the following major manifestations: carditis, migratory polyarthritis, chorea, erythema marginatum, and subcutaneous nodules. He has 3 of the 5 major criteria. Additionally, he has fever and evidence of recent Group A *Streptococcus* infection with the positive ASO titer. Even if *Streptococcus pyogenes* cannot be isolated, you still treat with a therapeutic course of 1.2 million units of IM penicillin as 1 dose or oral penicillin for 10 days. Most authorities recommend the IM injection in the setting of acute rheumatic fever. He would then go on prophylactic penicillin q month to prevent recurrent attacks. Steroids are not indicated for treatment of the arthritis. The arthritis will usually respond quite well to aspirin. However, many believe that there is a role for steroids in patients with severe carditis accompanied by congestive heart failure. But, neither salicylates nor glucocorticoids influence the future development of valvular heart disease. In adults, prednisone can be started in doses as high as 30 mg 4 times daily in especially severe cases; and as the patient improves, salicylates can be added during the tapering of the steroid dose; this may require 4 to 6 weeks.

Board Testing Point: Recognize the clinical criteria for rheumatic fever.

155. Answer: A

Answer: Infection transmitted by a bite from a tick.
His picture is consistent with manifestations of Lyme disease, which is transmitted by the bite of an *Ixodes scapularis* (formerly *I. dammini*). Lyme disease is due to *Borrelia burgdorferi*. His exposure occurred while he was "moonlighting" off Long Island, which is a high-risk area for Lyme disease. Lyme carditis is most often manifested by AV nodal conduction disturbances, anywhere from 1st through 3rd degree heart block. Treatment consists of a 3rd generation cephalosporin or doxycycline. It will usually resolve with treatment.

Cocaine can cause myocardial ischemia and infarction; but we have no evidence on ECG that this has occurred and his symptoms have been prolonged now for a while, so the ECG should have some evidence of damage at this point. HIV carditis would not present this way, and a coronary artery embolus would not present in this fashion over several days.

Board Testing Point: Recognize the clinical manifestations of Lyme disease carditis.

156. Answer: B

Answer: PVCs such as these can cause symptoms.
Palpitations are the most common symptoms that people will perceive from them. Symptoms can also occur if the stroke volume is decreased by decreasing overall ventricular filling. PVCs are common and occur in nearly 60% of men who undergo Holter monitoring. In patients who have known coronary artery disease, the frequency and nature of the PVCs do matter; generally, > 30/hour is associated with increased mortality. PVCs increase in frequency with aging, not decrease.

Board Testing Point: Recognize that even benign PVCs can be symptomatic but, in general, cause no harm.

157. Answer: B

Answer: Placement of a temporary pacing wire, and stop her diltiazem and atenolol.
The patient has significant symptomatic bradycardia with spells of sinus arrest. This is most likely due to her medications, particularly the beta-blocker. Elderly patients can be particularly at risk for AV nodal blockade from beta-blockers and diltiazem, especially when used in combination. Thus, we could probably temporarily pace her and then see if the bradycardia resolves off the medications. She is symptomatic and has significant pauses, so just stopping the medication alone would not be correct; a temporary pacer is needed at this point. Using atropine would not be effective for prolonged periods of time if this were drug-induced; plus, it is likely to cause her more harm.

Board Testing Point: Recognize symptomatic bradycardia and the need for temporary pacing in a patient who needs urgent surgery.

158. Answer: E

Answer: Hypertrophic cardiomyopathy (idiopathic hypertropic subaortic stenosis).
He has all of the classic findings of hypertropic cardiomyopathy. He has a harsh systolic murmur without radiation to the neck. The murmur is due to the intracavitary obstruction in the left ventricle. The murmur increases with Valsalva or any other maneuver that will decrease left ventricular size, which will increase the outflow obstruction and the intensity of the murmur. Conversely, maneuvers that increase left ventricular blood volume (squatting and passive leg-raising) will "move" the muscular obstruction protruding into the outflow track away from the opposite wall, decreasing the obstruction and the murmur. The brisk carotid upstroke is also part of this condition. Additionally, the history was helpful; the death of his older brother suggests the "familial" form of this disease.

Board Testing Point: Recognize the clinical manifestations of hypertrophic cardiomyopathy.

159. Answer: B

Answer: Echocardiogram.
This patient has hypertrophic cardiomyopathy. All aspects of his physical examination correlate with this diagnosis: The harsh systolic murmur that does not radiate to the neck increases with standing and decreases with squatting. The history of his brother dying of "sudden" death supports the familial form of this disease and increased risk for sudden cardiac death. An echocardiogram is diagnostic test of choice and will show you the asymmetric septal hyperthrophy with small left ventricular cavity and systolic anterior motion of the mitral valve. A treadmill stress test (blood pressure response) and Holter monitor (prolonged or repetitive episodes of nonsustained ventricular tachycardia) are often done as a part of risk stratification to estimate risk for sudden cardiac death; however, neither will confirm diagnosis. The ECG can be suggestive of hypertrophic cardiomyopathy. It may show Q waves in the inferior to lateral leads (from the hypertrophied septum) and have a normal-to-increased voltage (depending on the degree of LVH) with anterolateral T wave inversions consistent with repolarization abnormality. Athletes with HCM (with or without obstruction) should not participate in competitive sports.

Board Testing Point: Be able to diagnose hypertrophic cardiomyopathy.

160. Answer: A

Answer: Thrombolytics for treatment of an acute MI.
This patient has acute pericarditis by his symptoms and physical examination. It is very unlikely that this healthy young man has had an MI. Diffuse concave-up ST elevation is seen with pericarditis, as opposed to localized concave-down ST elevation seen in an acute MI. Everything else listed you would do for symptomatic relief. Admission is warranted to follow his course and look for common etiologies, although it is likely that this will be idiopathic after his viral infection. Finally, thrombolytics in this setting is not only wrong (there is no MI) but could cause a hemorrhagic pericardial effusion and tamponade.

Board Testing Point: Recognize the clinical findings of pericarditis and its treatment.

161. Answer: D

Answer: Holter study.
She likely is having an arrhythmia (such as SVT) from her caffeine intake. The best test would be to monitor on a Holter and then see which arrhythmia is occurring. The other tests are not indicated at this time.

Board Testing Point: Recognize that Holter monitor is the best study to evaluate palpitations without other signs or symptoms.

162. Answer: D

Answer: Dobutamine stress echo.
This patient is diabetic and has some symptoms suggestive of coronary artery disease. He cannot perform a routine stress test due to his arthritis. An electrophysiologic study is not going to tell us anything. This could be an ulcer, but the pressing issue is whether or not he has coronary artery disease. Proceeding to left heart catheterization is invasive and not necessary at this point. Pharmacological type of stress test (dobutamine stress echo or adenosine/regadenoson nuclear stress test) should be helpful in determining if he has significant coronary disease—if so, then a left heart cath would be indicated.

Board Testing Point: Understand how to work up coronary artery disease in a patient who cannot walk on a standard treadmill.

163. Answer: C

Answer: Starting nitroprusside or nitroglycerin IV for afterload reduction.
That would be the **1** thing here you would **not** want to do. His blood pressure is already low, and he is in cardiogenic shock. You do not want afterload reduction—this will make his hypotension acutely worse. All of the other choices are appropriate, depending on the hospital setting you are in. Obviously, if a cath lab was not available, management should include fibrinolytic therapy, inotropic agents, and placement of an intraaortic ballon pump (if possible), followed by immediate transfer to a PCI (percutaneous coronary intervention) facility.

Board Testing Point: Recognize the appropriate management of a hemodynamically unstable acute MI.

164. Answer: D

Answer: Schedule surgery in 3 months, if clinically unchanged.
In the majority of cardiac patients having noncardiac surgery, the highest potential risk is from coronary artery disease. In this patient with a history of recent MI, the incidence of reinfarction during a major noncardiac surgery averages approximately 6%. The risk, however, is inversely proportional to the time since the MI. For example, within the first 3 months the risk is 37%; after 6 months, it falls to 4–5%. In this patient, it would be better to wait another 3 months before doing this elective surgery. Additionally, he is having exercise testing daily with his skating to work for 3 miles and his lawn mowing on the weekend. Studies have shown that an exercise capacity of 5–6 METs indicates that cardiac risk during noncardiac surgery is low. Mowing the lawn easily reaches this threshold; therefore, formal testing is not indicated and is just an added expense.

Board Testing Point: Understand that most elective non-cardiac surgery may occur safely 6 months after a previous MI.

165. Answer: D

Answer: Vascular surgery consultation for aneurysm repair.
In 2005, the ACC/AHA guidelines were published. She has an infrarenal abdominal aortic aneurysm (AAA) that has surpassed the threshold level of 5.5 cm. Below 4 cm, these aneurysms are low-risk for rupture. Between 4 to 5.4 cm, infrarenal or juxtarenal AAAs should be monitored by ultrasound/CT every 6–12 months to detect expansion. In those with AAAs smaller than 4.0 cm, most recommend ultrasound monitoring every 2–3 years. Intervention is not recommended for asymptomatic infrarenal or juxtarenal AAAs if they measure < 5 cm for men and < 4.5 cm for women. In this case, now that she has been found to have a 5.6-cm aneurysm, the best choice is to proceed with surgery.

Board Testing Point: Know the ACC/AHA practice guidelines for aortic aneurysm repair.

166. Answer: B

Answer: Notify your cardiovascular surgeon to come right away and evaluate her for emergent mitral valve replacement.
She has likely had a papillary muscle rupture and developed acute mitral insufficiency. The murmur is classically a holosystolic murmur at the apex, as opposed to being located at the left sternal border with acute ventricular septal defects. Pericardiocentesis is not indicated, because she has no evidence indicating tamponade, which you would see with a left ventricular free wall rupture. The lack of syncope also points more toward ruptured papillary muscle instead of ventricular septum rupture or left ventricular free wall rupture.

Board Testing Point: Recognize the clinical features of papillary muscle rupture after an MI.

167. Answer: D

Answer: History of previous endocarditis.
This would indicate significant risk for recurrent endocarditis. The other items are low-risk and do not require prophylaxis. In 2007, new AHA guidelines were published and essentially eliminated all indications for prophylaxis except for these:

- Prosthetic heart valves, including bioprosthetic and homograft valves
- Prosthetic material used for cardiac valve repair
- A prior history of infective endocarditis
- Unrepaired cyanotic congenital heart disease, including palliative shunts and conduits
- Completely repaired congenital heart defects with prosthetic material or device, whether placed by surgery or by catheter intervention, during the first 6 months after the procedure
- Repaired congenital heart disease with residual defects at the site or adjacent to the site of the prosthetic device
- Cardiac "valvulopathy" in a transplanted heart

Common valvular lesions for which antimicrobial prophylaxis is no longer recommended in the 2007 AHA guidelines include bicuspid aortic valve, acquired aortic or mitral valve disease (including mitral valve prolapse with regurgitation and those who have undergone prior valve repair), and hypertrophic cardiomyopathy with latent or resting obstruction. Additionally, only certain dental procedures that cause perforation of oral mucosa or involve gingival manipulation (routine cleaning is okay), respiratory tract procedures, or skin/musculoskeletal tissue (if staphylococci or beta-hemolytic streptococci are likely) procedures require prophylaxis; genitourinary or gastrointestinal procedures no longer require prophylaxis.

Board Testing Point: Know the latest endocarditis prophylaxis guidelines.

168. Answer: E

Answer: None of these choices requires prophylaxis.
In 2007, new AHA guidelines were published and essentially eliminated all indications for prophylaxis except for these:

- Prosthetic heart valves, including bioprosthetic and homograft valves
- Prosthetic material used for cardiac valve repair
- A prior history of infective endocarditis
- Unrepaired cyanotic congenital heart disease, including palliative shunts and conduits
- Completely repaired congenital heart defects with prosthetic material or device, whether placed by surgery or by catheter intervention, during the first 6 months after the procedure
- Repaired congenital heart disease with residual defects at the site or adjacent to the site of the prosthetic device
- Cardiac "valvulopathy" in a transplanted heart

Common valvular lesions for which antimicrobial prophylaxis is no longer recommended in the 2007 AHA guidelines include bicuspid aortic valve, acquired aortic or mitral valve disease (including mitral valve prolapse with regurgitation and those who have undergone prior valve repair), and hypertrophic cardiomyopathy with latent or resting obstruction. Additionally, only certain dental procedures that cause perforation of oral mucosa or involve gingival manipulation (routine cleaning is okay), respiratory tract procedures, or skin/musculoskeletal tissue (if staphylococci or beta-hemolytic streptococci are likely) procedures require prophylaxis; genitourinary or gastrointestinal procedures no longer require prophylaxis.

Board Testing Point: Know the latest endocarditis prophylaxis guidelines. (We include these guidelines more than once to underscore the importance of knowing them.)

169. Answer: D

Answer: No, presence of prosthetic joints does not require antibiotic prophylaxis.
There is some controversy about the use of antibiotic prophylaxis for prolonged surgery or surgery involving infected areas—but some authorities do recommend prophylaxis. But for routine dental procedures, no prophylaxis is indicated. Remember: She has anaphylaxis to penicillin—you certainly would not use amoxicillin, and you would be a little leery of using a cephalosporin too.

Board Testing Point: Recognize that for routine dental procedures antibiotic prophylaxis is not recommended for patients who have prosthetic joints.

170. Answer: A

Answer: Hypertrophic obstructive cardiomyopathy (HOCM).
The combination of:

1) "spike and dome" carotid pulse contour,
2) similar apex cardiogram,
3) holosystolic murmur,
4) murmur augmentation by standing,
5) murmur augmentation by Valsalva strain,
6) the Brockenbrough phenomenon (premature contractions followed by diminished radial artery impulses), and
7) sudden death (resuscitated)

makes the diagnosis of hypertrophic (obstructive) cardiomyopathy inescapable here. The pure form of this disease is now known to be an autosomal dominant transmission, thus explaining the importance of investigating other members of the kindred, particularly in the type of scenario described. This entity is 1 of the several diagnoses that is customarily first considered when there is an acute event in an elite athlete. Other entities worth consideration in this regard are WPW, Marfan physiology, anomalous coronary disease, and long QT_c syndrome.

Appropriate associations with the other entities mentioned might include:

- Myxomatous mitral valve prolapse (MVP): mid-systolic click
- Ostium secundum atrial septal defect (ASD): fixed splitting of S_2
- Ostium primum atrioventricular septal defect (AVSD): RBBB/LAFB
- Acquired (muscular) ventricular septal defect (VSD): myocardial infarction
- Wolff-Parkinson-White syndrome (WPW): delta waves
- Congenital long QT syndrome: $QT_c > 0.43–0.44$

Board Testing Point: Recognize the clinical findings of hypertrophic obstructive cardiomyopathy.

171. Answer: A

Answer: Mural thrombus formation on a ruptured or eroded atherosclerotic plaque.
During the past 20 years, we have learned an enormous amount about the pathogenesis and treatment of unstable angina. In most cases of unstable rest angina, the pathogenesis is a mural thrombus formation on a ruptured or eroded atherosclerotic plaque. All of the other factors are legitimate entities, and could even be operative in this particular patient, but the key to a correct answer is the most likely concept, rather than attempting to focus on lesser issues.

Board Testing Point: Recognize that the etiology of acute unstable angina is most likely a thrombus formation on a ruptured or eroded atherosclerotic plaque.

172. Answer: C

Answer: Urgent revascularization.
The prognosis for the patient with cardiogenic shock in the setting of myocardial infarction is limited and is a function of the amount of lost myocardium. The threshold value is usually stated to be 40%; losses above that amount generally are those that account for shock. The patient with acute papillary muscle disruption or perforation of the interventricular septum represents special, uniquely surgical challenges. The patient described here used to be seen as nearly hopeless until the observation that some may improve dramatically if given a successful catheter revascularization approach. Getting her to the cath lab as quickly as possible is the best chance for recovering/maintaining viable myocardium. If the cath lab is not available (e.g., rural community), then fibrinolytics are indicated.

Board Testing Point: Recognize that in the setting of an acute anterior MI with Q waves, immediate/urgent revascularization in the cath lab is the best choice.

173. Answer: C

Answer: Tricuspid regurgitation.
The patients of this nature are so familiar in some geographic settings that the diagnosis is nearly routine. The characteristic features of tricuspid regurgitation accompanied by septic pulmonary emboli and evidence of parenteral drug usage predict that *Staphylococcus aureus* will be isolated as the causative agent in the majority of cases. Some of these patients have even had their tricuspid valves removed rather than attempting to implant a prosthetic device in a patient who could return to bacteremia-associated behaviors (via relapse). This is something that can be done if the patient has no additional heart disease. An alternative to this approach might include a plastic repair of the native valve, a so-called "vegetectomy."

Board Testing Point: Recognize the clinical manifestations of tricuspid regurgitation in the setting of IV drug abuse.

174. Answer: C

Answer: Biventricular congestive heart failure.
The key to the correct answer here is the noting of left ventricular gallop rhythm and pulmonary edema, thereby implicating **left** heart failure, as well as right. Acute pulmonary thromboembolism represents, effectively, **acute** cor pulmonale. Normally, we think of chronic cor pulmonale heart disease occurring in the COPD-type patient (e.g., the "blue bloater" patient with chronic bronchitis). The choice of pericardial effusion with pericardial tamponade would be unacceptable for the same reason (e.g., failing to account for the left heart failure), but also because there are no data per se presented to support a diagnosis of pericardial disease.

Eisenmenger transformation requires a shunt lesion, which is not there; this patient is most often a young adult with a large ventricular septal defect whose torrential left-to-right shunting is converted, at least to a balanced shunting phenomenon, if not an actual reversal to right-to-left shunting.

Board Testing Point: Recognize the clinical manifestations of biventricular congestive heart failure.

175. Answer: E

Answer: Pericardiocentesis.
Clinical presentation is consistent with hemodynamically significant pericardial tamponade (hypotension, tachycardia, distended neck veins with prominent "x" descent, globular cardiac silhouette and the presence of pulsus paradoxus). The treatment principles in this setting include the following:

1) Positive inotropic support
2) (Rapid) Volume infusion
3) Pericardiocentesis under controlled circumstances
4) Pericardiostomy

Patients with pericardial tamponade are preload dependent so they should not receive IV furosemide (as this will drop blood pressure even more!), and because of the possibility that this could be a hemorrhagic effusion, thrombolytics are contraindicated, as they could worsen the effusion (more bleeding!).

Board Testing Point: Recognize the clinical manifestations of cardiac tamponade, and know its treatment and diagnostic management.

176. Answer: A

Answer: Myxomatous mitral valve prolapse (MVP).
Auscultatory findings are consistent with mitral valve prolapse. Augmentation of murmur with standing and Valsalva strain exclude ASD, AVSD and VSD, and presence of mid-systolic click favors MVP in comparison to HOCM. In addition, the murmur of HOCM gets softer with handgrip.

Board Testing Point: Recognize the cardiac findings of mitral valve prolapse.

177. Answer: C

Answer: Cor pulmonale due to pulmonary thromboembolism.
It is very important to appreciate the fact that **acute** cor pulmonale represents pulmonary thromboembolism almost by definition. This gentleman may represent another variation on the so-called "economy class syndrome" theme that has been a concern in the commercial air transportation community, although the nature of the association, if any, remains uncertain. Of far more importance in this particular patient may be the neoplasm, the association between a true hypercoagulable state and known cancer. This patient has all the features of (acute) pulmonary hypertension and right heart failure. The systemic venous hypertension, as reflected in his jugular venous pulsations, reminds us of the differential diagnosis of this physical finding, which is:

1) Right heart failure
2) Tricuspid valve disease
3) Pericardial compressive physiology
4) Superior vena cava syndrome

Note that the patient with superior vena cava syndrome would have distended, pulseless neck veins as well as the other features that so often accompany the Pancoast tumor—e.g., Horner syndrome, collar of Stokes, facial suffusion, and a characteristic chest x-ray.

Board Testing Point: Recognize the clinical manifestations of pulmonary thromboembolism in a patient with multiple risk factors.

---

178. Answer: A

Answer: Normal repolarization variant.
Early repolarization (ER), also known as benign early repolarization (BER) or normal variant, is noted in approximately 1% to 2% of the population and in up to 48% of patients with chest pain who are seen in the emergency department. The electrocardiographic characteristics of ER include widespread ST-segment elevation, upward concavity of the initial portion of the ST segment, notching of the terminal QRS complex, and concordant T waves of large amplitude. The incidence of 1% to 2% is found equally common in all races. The findings are known to regress during exercise testing. The nearly universal impression of an increased frequency in African-American men is not well documented in the literature, although there are very thoughtful statements as to the significance with respect to both thrombolysis criteria and cocaine usage. This patient's chest pain may be GI (stress → GERD), as well as anxiety over the case he is working on.

Board Testing Point: Understand the concept of a normal repolarization variant in a young person.

---

179. Answer: B

Answer: Pulmonary arterial hypertension, acquired via cor pulmonale.
In contrast to the patient with pulmonary thromboembolism and **acute** cor pulmonale, here is the typical picture of **chronic** cor pulmonale heart disease in the setting of what is no doubt chronic bronchitis. This is the traditional association of the classic "blue bloater" and the development of pulmonary hypertension, no doubt as a function of the chronic arterial hypoxemia for which they are so well known, although the mechanism is the same in cystic fibrosis.

Board Testing Point: Recognize the clinical features of cor pulmonale and its resulting heart disease.

---

180. Answer: D

Answer: Ventricular tachycardia (VT).
From a test-taker's point of view, there are **8 key points** in this case, as follows:

1) Older adult
2) Alcohol
3) Syncope
4) Tachycardia at a rate of about 150/min
5) Regular rhythm
6) **Wide** QRS complexes
7) Atrioventricular dissociation
8) Ventricular rate greater than atrial rate

With that data base, one is searching for the answer that fits the ECG criteria, which is sufficient to cause syncope, and which the patient could survive long enough to permit the depiction shared by the paramedics. As such, ventricular tachycardia can be the only answer. No one "regains consciousness" during ventricular fibrillation. AV dissociation excludes AV nodal reentry tachycardia and sinus tachycardia. Multifocal atrial tachycardia is not regular.

This question in particular is included to demonstrate the process of diagnostic clinical reasoning. The association with alcohol intake is well documented.

Board Testing Point: Recognize the clinical characteristics associated with ventricular tachycardia.

---

181. Answer: A

Answer: Ostium secundum atrial septal defect (ASD).
The fixed splitting of the 2nd heart sound points you to the single best answer. The flow murmur is typical and represents the shunt volume in the pulmonary artery. In fact, there may be a murmur resulting from the flow across the septal defect itself, but this is a diastolic murmur and is seldom heard clinically.

This phenomenon is also largely exhalation-dependent and is, therefore, exactly what explains the fixed splitting: Whereas **inspiration** volume loads the right ventricle in the usual fashion (via acceleration of caval flow), **expiration** volume loads the right ventricle again (via the increase in shunt volume across the septal defect itself in exhalation), thereby resulting in a balance of loading phenomena affecting the right heart (and effectively "holding" P_2 away from A_2).

Board Testing Point: Recognize the clinical findings of an ASD.

---

182. Answer: D

Answer: Coarctation of the aorta.
The equality of the upper limbs and disparity of the upper versus lower limbs helps identify a narrowing beyond the left subclavian artery.

Board Testing Point: Recognize the clinical features of coarctation of the aorta.

---

183. Answer: E

Answer: A ventilation/perfusion lung scan showing multiple perfusion defects.
The woman has infective endocarditis of the tricuspid valve, a common occurrence in intravenous drug users. An echocardiogram would be very likely to show a tricuspid vegetation. Given her symptoms and the lung findings, she almost certainly has multiple septic emboli to the lungs, a problem that would be best identified by a ventilation/perfusion lung scan. She has several signs of right heart failure and pulmonary hypertension, but no signs of left heart failure. All of the other choices would reflect left heart failure.

She will need intravenous antibiotics for an extended period of time, and possibly tricuspid valve removal. Some patients do fairly well without a tricuspid valve, but others have refractory peripheral edema, liver congestion, ascites, and so forth. They may require tricuspid valve replacement, usually with a bioprosthetic valve, since mechanical valves have a high thrombosis rate in the tricuspid position. Clearly, any prosthetic valve in an IV drug abuser is subject to reinfection.

High resolution CT of the chest can also be used to distinguish pulmonary septic emboli from TV endocarditis.

Board Testing Point: Recognize the clinical features of an IV-drug abuser with suspected endocarditis.

184. Answer: C

Answer: Hypertrophic cardiomyopathy.
There has been heightened awareness of sudden death of young people partaking in strenuous exercise after several highly publicized cases. The largest series of autopsies in these individuals have shown no abnormalities in the majority of patients. Death was presumably due to a ventricular arrhythmia from an unrecognized source, possibly a subclinical cardiomyopathy or an unknown genetic disorder. If any abnormality is found on autopsy, hypertrophic cardiomyopathy is the most common, followed by anomalous origin of the coronary arteries.

Board Testing Point: Know that at autopsy for sudden death, usually no abnormalities are found; but if an abnormality is found, the most common is hypertrophic cardiomyopathy.

185. Answer: C

Answer: A sound heard with the diaphragm at the apex shortly after S_2.
The woman has rheumatic mitral stenosis. Mitral stenosis would likely be an opening snap heard at the apex after S_2. The opening snap is a high-pitched sound, and thus heard better with the diaphragm. Scarlet fever is caused by a group A strep (GAS) infection, which can cause acute rheumatic fever (ARF). Rheumatic heart disease develops over a period of years after 1 or more bouts of untreated ARF. Mitral stenosis is a common finding that can occur anywhere from 5 to 20 years later.

S_1 is typically loud in mitral stenosis. Aortic regurgitation would produce a decrescendo blowing murmur at the left lower sternal border with the patient sitting forward. Mitral valve prolapse would present with the click and murmur. A sound heard with the bell at the apex after S_2 would be an S_3, which patients with mitral stenosis are very unlikely to have, since the left ventricle is not filled rapidly.

Board Testing Point: Recognize the physical exam features of mitral stenosis.

186. Answer: B

Answer: Large *a* waves and very large *v* waves.
This person has advanced left and right heart failure from previous myocardial infarctions. Large *a* and *v* waves would be typical of this condition. Large *a* waves and slow *y* descents are associated with tricuspid stenosis. Rapid *x* and *y* descents are found in constrictive pericarditis. A cannon *a* wave occurs with atrio-ventricular dissociation and RA contraction against a closed tricuspid valve (found in ventricular tachycardia). Distended non-pulsatile neck veins would be indicative of superior vena caval obstruction, most likely from cancer.

Board Testing Point: Be familiar with wave formations in the neck.

187. Answer: E

Answer: Acute mitral regurgitation from rupture of a myxomatous chordae.
The patient has acute severe mitral regurgitation from rupture of a myxomatous chordae of the mitral valve. The clues are the sudden onset of symptoms in an otherwise healthy middle-aged man, the prominent apical impulse (which means this is **not** a left ventricular function problem), and the early systolic decrescendo murmur. Unilateral opacification on a chest x-ray is an uncommon but well-reported presentation of pulmonary edema.

There is no evidence of a myocardial infarction, particularly with the impressive apical impulse and normal electrocardiogram. There cannot be a new VSD because the murmur would be hard to miss and, again, he has no evidence of an acute infarction. Acute aortic regurgitation could present exactly like this, except that it should produce an early diastolic murmur. Transesophageal echo, had it been available, would easily have made the correct diagnosis, since the echo image would be unaffected by his mechanical ventilation.

Board Testing Point: Recognize the clinical features of acute mitral regurgitation from rupture of a myxomatous chordae.

188. Answer: B

Answer: Transfer him emergently for mitral valve repair or replacement.
This man needs urgent cardiothoracic surgical intervention for the mitral valve. His mortality risk without immediate surgery is obviously very high. The other choices either are for incorrect diagnoses or delayed mitral valve surgery.

Board Testing Point: Recommend emergent surgical management for acute mitral regurgitation.

189. Answer: A

Answer: Prescribe sublingual nitroglycerin as needed and begin secondary prevention for coronary artery disease.
This man clearly has coronary artery disease. However, it takes an almost heroic amount of exercise to induce symptoms and evidence of ischemia. His exercise results, particularly his long duration of exercise, risk-stratify him by the Duke criteria to a 0.25% one-year cardiac mortality. He should receive aggressive secondary prevention, which has a very good chance of making him asymptomatic as well.

He certainly does not need immediate catheterization and revascularization based on his noninvasive test results. Amlodipine is a reasonable choice for treating his hypertension, but it is not part of standard secondary prevention that includes the antihypertensive beta-blockers. There is no need to spend money to obtain further validation of his ischemic heart disease by ordering thallium scintigraphy. Sublingual nitroglycerin is appropriate, but initial therapy with an angiotensin-converting enzyme inhibitor is not part of standard secondary prevention. He has no evidence of left heart failure that would justify the use of this medication.

Board Testing Point: Recommend therapy for a patient with excellent exercise capacity and presumed coronary artery disease.

190. Answer: D

Answer: A ventilation/perfusion lung scan.
This complex patient turned out to have normal coronary arteries and pulmonary hypertension. His chronically edematous leg is the source of multiple pulmonary emboli. There is typically a 10-month delay between the onset of symptoms until the diagnosis is made, and then only when the patient has advanced pulmonary hypertension. The treatment of this condition was nearly hopeless until pulmonary thromboendarterectomy was developed.

Any type of echocardiogram would show right heart enlargement and pulmonary hypertension, but the latter is obvious from the hemodynamic data. An arterial blood gas might demonstrate hypoxia, but would certainly not be diagnostic. The DLCO would be abnormal, but not specific.

Board Testing Point: Know that unrecognized pulmonary embolisms can result in an insidious presentation for pulmonary hypertension.

191. Answer: A

Answer: Patient A is more likely than patient B to have pulsus paradoxus.
These hemodynamic tracings are from patients with tamponade (A) and constrictive pericarditis (B). The only one of the choices that would be expected with tamponade is pulsus paradoxus. The other findings are typical of constriction.

Board Testing Point: Recognize the hemodynamic differences between constrictive pericorditis and tamponade.

192. Answer: E

Answer: Treat the immediate pain with an intravenous narcotic and start ibuprofen 2,400 mg/day.
This woman has atypical chest pain for ischemia and an electrocardiogram that shows diffuse ST-segment elevation and PR-segment depression, most prominent in lead II. This is the classic ECG for acute pericarditis and should be treated with pain medications and nonsteroidal antiinflammatory agents. The worst possible course would be to give thrombolytic therapy, which could result in acute bleeding from the inflamed pericardium and subsequent tamponade.

Board Testing Point: Recognize the clinical findings and treatment of acute pericarditis.

193. Answer: C

Answer: A 75-year-old man with the onset of chest pain 5 hours ago and a new left bundle-branch block.
Patients with new left bundle-branch block in the clinical setting of an acute ischemic event have the most mortality benefit from thrombolytic therapy because of the amount of myocardium in jeopardy. Patients with anterior ST-segment elevation benefit less, with inferior ST-segment elevation still less, and are actually harmed with ST-segment depression. The 80-year-old woman has a strong indication for thrombolytic therapy, except for the recent onset of a neurological deficit. The 72-year-old woman with a tall R wave in leads V1 and V2 is having an acute posterior MI and would benefit from thrombolytic therapy to the same extent as an acute inferior MI.

Board Testing Point: Recognize that patients with larger areas of potential left ventricular ischemia (e.g., left bundle-branch block) will benefit the most from immediate reperfusion.

194. Answer: B

Answer: A large, lobulated, mobile mass in the apex of the left ventricle.
This poor man had a recent large myocardial infarction and suffered a severe complication. All of the findings point to a severe metabolic acidosis, probably from mesenteric infarction from an arterial embolism from the apical thrombus.

His normal blood pressure alone rules out cardiogenic shock, acute mitral regurgitation, acute ventricular septal defect, and free-wall rupture—the 4 causes of sudden shock after myocardial infarction.

Board Testing Point: Recognize the clinical findings of an arterial embolism.

---

195. Answer: E

Answer: Aortic dissection can occur in the 3rd trimester of pregnancy without any obvious predisposing factors.

Aortic dissections that involve the ascending aorta should always be treated surgically. Appropriate medical therapy is both beta-blockers and nitroprusside. The hemodynamic parameter that is most associated with extension of the dissection is the rate of rise of the aortic pressure. Nitroprusside decreases the aortic systolic pressure, but actually increases the rate of rise because of reflex tachycardia. Beta-blockers and nitroprusside together decrease the rate of rise. Most descending thoracic dissections can be treated medically. Aortic dissection is an uncommon complication of pregnancy, usually occurring in the 3rd trimester. Dissection of the coronary arteries may also occur in pregnant women.

Board Testing Point: Recognize that aortic dissection can occur in the 3rd trimester of pregnancy without any predisposing factors.

---

196. Answer: A

Answer: Sudden cessation of the narrow QRS complex tachycardia followed by a 15-second period of asystole.

This man has the classic tachycardia-bradycardia syndrome in which a tachyarrhythmia, in this case the common form of PSVT (producing the regular cannon *a* waves in the neck), stops suddenly as a good reentrant arrhythmia should, and a long pause occurs before the sinus node begins capturing the atrium properly. Careful electrophysiological studies have shown that most of these pauses are caused by SA exit block; that is, the SA node is firing properly but not capturing the atrium. This occurs because of senile infiltration of the conduction system by fibrous tissue, the same cause of most AV nodal and bundle-branch blocks. The fibrous tissue is rendered refractory by a supraventricular tachycardia, most frequently atrial fibrillation and atrial flutter, and the patient experiences a long pause that can produce fainting. Treatment involves permanent pacemaker implantation to protect against the bradyarrhythmia, and then whatever treatment is appropriate for the tachyarrhythmia.

There is no reason why this man, without evidence of structural heart disease, should have ventricular tachycardia. Third-degree AV block would be unlikely to occur suddenly upon termination of a supraventricular tachycardia. There is no reason to suspect *torsade de pointes*. An atrial rate of 330 bpm is very fast for atrial flutter, and this rhythm would not produce regular cannon *a* waves.

Board Testing Point: Recognize the clinical characteristics of tachycardia-bradycardia syndrome.

---

197. Answer: C

Answer: Concentric left ventricular hypertrophy and a left ventricular ejection fraction of 80%.
This case represents a common misunderstanding of the hemodynamics of heart failure. This man has severe hypertension but is being treated incorrectly. His chest x-ray indicates that he has a large heart and a high pulmonary capillary wedge pressure, but it does not explain the underlying pathophysiology. He has diastolic dysfunction because of the stiffness of his hypertrophied ventricle, but nothing about the physical examination suggests left heart systolic dysfunction or valvular heart disease. He has a prominent apical impulse, indicating an actively contracting left ventricle, and a 4th heart sound caused by his high left ventricular end-diastolic pressure. If the proper therapy is not used, he will eventually end up with poor left ventricular function.

Board Testing Point: Understand the clinical manifestations of left ventricular hypertrophy without initial systolic dysfunction.

198. Answer: A

Answer: Stop digoxin, decrease the dose of furosemide, and start beta-blockers.
This man needs negative inotropic therapy with beta-blockers or verapamil. He may need some diuretic, but not enough to produce volume depletion and postural hypotension, as in this patient. He would need the therapy "Continue digoxin and furosemide; add an angiotensin-converting enzyme inhibitor, low-dose carvedilol, and spironolactone" if he had poor left ventricular function. Digoxin has no place in the treatment of a patient with hyperdynamic left ventricular function.

The 2 intravenous inotropic agents are occasionally used for severe end-stage systolic heart failure, although they do not have a Class I recommendation for this use.

Board Testing Point: Recognize the appropriate therapy for hypertension with LVH and a hyperdynamic LV.

199. Answer: C

Answer: An electrophysiology study.
This woman's electrocardiogram shows a short PR interval and a delta wave in several leads, consistent with the Wolff-Parkinson-White (WPW) syndrome. The modern treatment of patients with symptomatic arrhythmias and WPW is electrophysiology-guided ablation of the accessory pathway.

There is no reason why an otherwise healthy young woman needs an echocardiogram or a chest x-ray. She has pseudo-Q waves in the inferior leads and a tall R wave in V1, suggesting an inferoposterior myocardial infarction, but these are simply the delta waves in those leads. She appears to have left ventricular hypertrophy also, but again, this finding is not specific with this electrocardiogram.

Board Testing Point: Recognize Wolff-Parkinson-White (WPW) syndrome and the need for electrophysiology study to evaluate for ablation.

200. Answer: A

Answer: Contrast chest CT scan.
This patient has acute onset of chest pain radiating down his arms. He has a high arched palate on physical exam and a vague family history of his father dying of a "heart attack" at home at the age of 45. This patient has Marfan syndrome and is experiencing an aortic dissection. The best test is either a transesophageal echo or a contrast chest CT scan. It is appropriate to follow this patient in the CCU and obtain cardiac enzymes, but before anything else is done, he should be evaluated for aortic dissection.

Board Testing Point: Recognize Marfan syndrome and the clinical association with aortic dissection.

201. Answer: A

Answer: Trimethoprim/sulfamethoxazole.
The combination of warfarin and TMP/SMX can be a very deadly one. It is the most common warfarin interaction leading to hospitalization in the U.S.

Amoxicillin, codeine, and cefixime do not interact with warfarin. Azithromycin only rarely causes an increase in INR in patients on warfarin.

Board Testing Point: Recognize the effect trimethoprim/sulfamethoxazole may have on warfarin metabolism.

202. Answer: B

Answer: Acetaminophen.
This patient developed an unexplained increase in her INR. All the choices are drugs that patients can get over the counter or may get from another provider and not report (OCP). The correct answer is acetaminophen, which can increase the INR with as little as 3 extra-strength tablets a day. In 1 crossover study, patients on warfarin who took 4 grams of acetaminophen a day had INRs 1.75x higher than a group on warfarin and not taking acetaminophen.

Board Testing Point: Recognize the drug interaction between acetaminophen and warfarin.

203. Answer: A

Answer: Gingko biloba.
Gingko biloba can increase hemorrhage risk in patients who take it. It can further increase the risk in anticoagulated patients. Another agent to avoid is St. John's wort, which may increase the metabolism of warfarin and, if a patient isn't monitored closely, could lead to under-anticoagulation.

Folate, cat's claw, and saw palmetto do not affect warfarin metabolism.

Board Testing Point: Recognize the drug interaction between gingko biloba and warfarin.

204. Answer: E

Answer: Warfarin administration.
Increased PT with a normal PTT and platelets usually indicate warfarin administration. Factor VII deficiency could do this also.

Board Testing Point: Be familiar with what causes an isolated increased PT.

205. Answer: B

Answer: CBC with platelet count, PT, PTT, and bleeding time.
Note that coagulation factor deficiencies are more likely to present with complications such as hemarthrosis. Platelet disorders usually present with mucosal bleeding and a history of bleeding with light trauma. Knowing what the PTT, PT, and platelet counts are will help guide the direction in which you need to proceed. If the PT alone is elevated, then you know you are dealing with a deficiency/inhibitor of Factor VII, vitamin K deficiency, or liver disease. If the PTT alone is elevated, then you could be dealing with deficiency/inhibitors of Factors VIII, IX, or XI, or inhibitor of XII (deficiency of Factor XII does not cause a bleeding diathesis), von Willebrand disease, or lupus anticoagulant. Abnormal bleeding time would indicate von Willebrand disease or a platelet abnormality.

Board Testing Point: Recognize the laboratory tests to order in the initial workup of a bleeding disorder.

INFECTIOUS DISEASE

206. Answer: D

Answer: Continuous suppressive therapy with valacyclovir is beneficial in decreasing risk of transmission to the uninfected sexual partner.
Most people who acquire genital herpes are in a new sexual relationship. To prevent transmitting the virus, individuals with genital HSV infection should abstain from sexual activity if lesions or prodromal symptoms are present. However, virus shedding continues in infected individuals, even when asymptomatic. It is estimated that up to 70% of the HSV-2 transmissions occur while the infected person is asymptomatic. Condom use decreases the risk of HSV-2 transmission by about 50%. Continued suppressive therapy with valacyclovir of symptomatic patients (500 mg qd) also significantly decreases the risk of transmission to uninfected partners. It also has been shown to decrease the frequency of recurrence and the severity of symptoms. There is no recommendation for prophylactic antiretroviral therapy for the uninfected partner.

Board Testing Point: Prevent transmission of genital herpes virus.

207. Answer: D

Answer: Guillain-Barré syndrome.
Guillain-Barré is the most common acute inflammatory polyneuropathy. It frequently is preceded by an upper respiratory infection and has been associated with *Campylobacter jejuni* infections—as well as EBV, CMV, HIV, mycoplasma, and Lyme disease. Symptoms include an **ascending** paralysis and **areflexia** caused by a segmental demyelination of the peripheral nerves. CSF examination is not necessary to make the diagnosis but may show an elevated protein with a disproportionately smaller increase in CSF WBCs. Nerve conduction studies show slowed conduction due to demyelination. Plasmapheresis is useful if it is begun early in the course.

Botulism causes a **descending** paralysis and begins with **cranial** nerve weakness manifested by dysphonia, dysphagia, diplopia, and blurred vision; this is followed by the muscle weakness and respiratory insufficiency. Poliomyelitis presents as meningeal symptoms, fever, and asymmetric paralysis. Tick paralysis occurs while the tick is attached and is due to a neurotoxin. It causes an ascending flaccid paralysis and ataxia. Rabies causes an encephalitis characterized by fever, hydrophobia, and agitation progressing to coma and death. It does not have the peripheral nerve findings depicted in this case presentation.

Board Testing Point: Recognize the clinical features of Guillain-Barré syndrome.

208. Answer: A

Answer: Parvovirus B19.
Parvovirus B19 infects red cell precursors in the marrow and causes an arrest in red cell maturation (at the pronormoblast stage) with a resultant hypoproliferative anemia and high erythropoeitin levels. Immunocompetent patients will generate an immune response that clears the virus in about a week, and thus hemoglobin levels drop only 1–2 grams, which often goes unnoticed. Patients with late-stage HIV infection are incapable of mounting an immune response to the virus and develop a chronic, often severe anemia. Treatment is with IVIG, which contains sufficient levels of antibody to the virus to erradicate the infection. Zidovudine could cause anemia, but the anemia resolves after stopping the agent. HTLV-1's hematologic effect is to cause a T-cell lymphoma/leukemia and not pure red cell aplasia. Inhaled pentamidine is poorly absorbed and rarely causes any systemic toxicity. *Campylobacter* causes severe diarrhea in HIV-infected persons, but not red cell aplasia. Anemia is a well known dose-dependent side effect of zidovudine, but it resolves after discontinuation.

Board Testing Point: Know the association between parvovirus B19 and red cell aplasia in HIV-infected individuals.

209. Answer: C

Answer: Blastomycosis.
The combination of lung mass, draining cutaneous lesion, and the finding of budding yeast should point you toward either blastomycosis or histoplasmosis, both of which are present in Arkansas. Blastomycosis has broad-based budding (4 Bs: blasto, broad, based, bud). *Coccidioides* is seen in the Southwest, but its tissue form is a spherule, not a budding yeast. Tuberculosis and lung cancer would not explain the yeast on skin biopsy. Treatment would be with oral itraconazole for 6–12 months. If she were severely ill, you would use amphotericin B.

Board Testing Point: Recognize the geography and clinical features of blastomycosis.

210. Answer: E

Answer: Itraconazole and its metabolites are below therapeutic levels.
Itraconazole is the drug of choice for histoplasmosis but has reduced absorption with reduced stomach acid from H_2blockers or proton pump inhibitors. When this patient was placed on ranitidine with his itraconazole, the itraconazole was likely not absorbed as well, which allowed his histoplasmosis to relapse, as evidenced by yeast in the blood. It is more likely that he is reactivating a prior yeast infection rather than acquiring a new one (e.g., *Cryptococcus* or *Candida krusei*). *Histoplasma capsulatum* is rarely resistant to the azoles. Yeast in the blood should never be considered a contaminant.

Board Testing Point: Recognize that itraconazole requires an acidic stomach environment for best absorption and therapeutic levels.

211. Answer: B

Answer: Parvovirus B19.

Her child had the classic childhood presentation of parvovirus B19 "fifth disease," with slapped cheeks and a serpiginous rash that worsens with heat or sun exposure. His mother has the classic adult manifestation with arthritis and joint findings. In immunompetent patients, it is a self-limited illness. There are only 3 populations that run into more trouble. Pregnant women have a higher risk of fetal loss and hydrops fetalis. HIV-infected persons develop a chronic red cell aplasia treatable by IVIG, and persons with chronic hemolysis (e.g., sickle cell disease) develop an acute red cell aplasia that, if supported with transfusions, resolves. Human herpesvirus 6 causes roseola in kids and may be responsible for pneumonia and meningitis in immunocompromised adults. Lyme disease starts with erythema migrans in the majority of persons infected with *Borrelia burgdorferi*, and the late arthritis is usually an asymmetric mono- or oligoarthritis. Disseminated gonorrhea would not be present in both a child and a mother.

Board Testing Point: Know the clinical features of parvovirus B19 infection in adults, particularly the association with small joint arthritic pain.

212. Answer: A

Answer: *Chlamydophila pneumoniae.*

The constellation of symptoms—chronic non-productive cough, low-grade fever, hyperemic sore throat, hoarseness—fit this infection. *C. psittaci* is a concern, **but** he has no hepatosplenomegaly; plus, most commonly this presents as fever of abrupt onset, pronounced headache, and dry cough in a patient with a recent history of bird exposure. Systemic manifestations are prominent with fever in all patients, rigors occurring in a majority, with sweats and myalgias in most patients. A combination of pneumonia with splenomegaly: Think *C. psittaci* or *Coxiella burnetii*! Also think about *Coxiella* if the case notes he delivered cows or some livestock. Recently, cats have been implicated with this infection—but there usually has to be contact with placentas for this. *S. pneumoniae* is unlikely to produce this prolonged gradual infection, and the patchy infiltrate goes against it somewhat. In addition, the case kept saying he had no chills—if you see "chills" and "rusty sputum," think of *S. pneumoniae*.

Board Testing Point: Recognize the clinical features of *Chlamydophila pneumoniae* in a young person.

213. Answer: D

Answer: Intravenous ampicillin.

This poor woman has bacteremia with *Listeria*, a gram-positive diphtheroid-like organism. Think of this organism if pregnancy is involved (especially in the 3rd trimester after week 30 or so) or with someone who eats a lot of goat or imported cheeses, particularly from Mexico, or is an immigrant living in California. Penicillin or ampicillin is the only effective treatment; none of the other antibiotics is effective. Gentamicin can be used for synergy. She is bacteremic, so you are not going to use oral penicillin or ampicillin for this type of infection. If she is penicillin-allergic, you could use trimethoprim/sulfamethoxazole, or you could desensitize her if she was seriously ill. Normally, if you hear about a diphtheroid-like organism you suspect contamination—however, in someone immunocompromised or semi-immunocompromised (like pregnancy), don't ignore the blood culture result until you are sure it comes back as something unimportant.

Board Testing Point: Know that, for *Listeria* bacteremia, IV penicillin or ampicillin is the drug of choice.

214. Answer: A

Answer: Treat with oral metronidazole.
In 2010, the Infectious Diseases Society of America (IDSA) updated the recommendations for the treatment of *C. difficile* infection. Mild-to-moderate disease should be treated with metronidazole and severe disease with vancomycin. With either therapy, approximately 25% will relapse. The IDSA recommends an initial relapse that is mild-to-moderate be treated again with metronidazole. Vancomycin does not have a higher cure rate than metronidazole, and a 10-day course is exceedingly more expensive than metronidazole (~ $1,000 vs. ~ $20).

Fidaxomicin was FDA-approved in 2011 for the treatment of *C. difficile* infection. It has a similar cure rate as that of vancomycin but a 50% reduction in relapses. It may be considered in patients with frequent relapses, but it is not indicated for use after only 1 relapse as in this case. It costs ~ $3,000 for a 10-day course.

Board Testing Point: Know that metronidazole is the current treatment of choice for mild-to-moderate *C. difficile* diarrhea and that if a relapse occurs, it is still the best agent to use.

215. Answer: B

Answer: Azithromycin weekly.
His CD4 count has fallen below 50, putting him at risk for *Mycobacterium avium* complex (MAC) infection. Of the choices listed, only the azithromycin weekly is currently approved for prophylaxis. Clarithromycin could be used, but he would have to take it daily. Rifampin is not approved for MAC prophylaxis. A rifabutin and clarithromycin combo would be used for treatment, not prophylaxis. The choice of "nothing" is not correct, because he really is at high risk for MAC infection.

Board Testing Point: Understand that with a CD4 cell count of below 50 you should prophylax for MAC—and that azithromycin weekly is the most commonly used agent for prophylaxis.

216. Answer: C

Answer: Ceftriaxone and vancomycin.
Based on the Gram stain, she has pneumococcal meningitis. Realize that in many parts of the United States up to 30% of pneumococci are resistant to penicillin, and up to 10% are resistant to the 3rd generation cephalosporins. Know that vancomycin and ceftriaxone are appropriate for presumed pneumococcal meningitis until the sensitivities are known. Her prior antibiotic usage increases her risk of having a beta-lactam resistant organism. Penicillin alone would be a poor choice because of the high resistance rates. Now, if they tell you the pneumococcus is sensitive to penicillin, then that would be the correct choice!

Board Testing Point: Presumed pneumococcal meningitis should be initially treated with vancomycin and ceftriaxone until sensitivities are available.

217. Answer: C

Answer: *Tropheryma whipplei.*
Patients will present after a **long** time with nonspecific complaints. The main symptoms are weight loss, diarrhea, and arthropathies—and in nearly 75% of the cases these 3 occur together. The GI symptoms usually begin later but frequently lead to the diagnosis. Usually, they will present with episodic and watery diarrhea or steatorrhea accompanied by abdominal pain and, in about 20–30%, they will have occult blood in their stool.

Skin hyperpigmentation is frequently common to the sun-exposed areas. Just about every organ in the body will be infected with this bacterium. The diagnosis is usually made by upper endoscopy, but biopsy of lymph nodes or masses will also yield the diagnosis. Upper endoscopy will show whitish or yellowish plaques distributed on a friable mucosa. The key here is the PAS staining. PCR is also now available and would be useful for confirming this diagnosis. With PAS staining, be careful, because a few other conditions in the colon or rectum would show you this—for example, melanosis coli. *Trophermyma whipplei* is best treated with trimethoprim/sulfamethoxazole, but severely ill patients like this guy should receive parenteral ceftriaxone initially for at least 2 weeks. Amazingly, chloramphenicol (that old antibiotic) would be a good consideration for CNS disease too because of its great penetration.

Board Testing Point: Know the clinical manifestations and laboratory features (PAS staining) of Whipple disease.

218. Answer: B

Answer: Disseminated *Histoplasma* infection.
Note that the patient has AIDS. She lives in Memphis, which is endemic for *Histoplasma.* We can rule out coccidioidomycosis based on her geography. Disseminated *Pneumocystis* is rare outside of the lung. Lymphoma is possible but less likely, given her other findings. Tuberculosis also would be less likely to cause this picture. If she had a higher CD4 count—of, say, 300—we would be more concerned about tuberculosis than an opportunistic infection like *Histoplasma.*

Back to the *Histoplasma.* She has disseminated disease. It is likely that if we did a bone marrow aspiration, we would find the organism there. Also, today we can do blood cultures and effectively grow the organism quite easily. The other simple test to do would be a serum or urine *Histoplasma* antigen. This is highly sensitive and specific for disseminated *Histoplasma* in HIV-infected patients.

Board Testing Point: Recognize the clinical findings of disseminated *Histoplasma* in a patient with HIV and low CD4 count in a geographically compatible region.

219. Answer: E

Answer: Herpes simplex meningoencephalitis.
The key here is the "bizarre behavior" and the findings on MRI of temporal lobe involvement. To help you diagnose this, a PCR for herpes simplex virus DNA could be helpful on the CSF. CSF cultures for herpes are rarely positive, except in the severely immunocompromised or in neonates. He certainly is at risk for syphilis, but neurosyphilis takes decades to occur and is rare in teenagers unless they are HIV-infected. You would, though, order a CSF VDRL on this patient just because he is at high risk based on his past history. *Bartonella henselae* is the etiology for cat-scratch disease (for which he has no exposure history) and does cause significant CNS disease on occasion; usually it will present with seizures, which is likely with herpes encephalitis too. He has no rash consistent with varicella, and this does not look like bacterial meningitis with the normal protein and glucose.

Board Testing Point: Recognize the clinical features of herpes meningoencephalitis.

220. Answer: C

Answer: Sucralfate.
This agent will substantially interfere with the absorption of the oral drug, resulting in subtherapeutic serum and urine levels. Other agents to avoid that also will do this include antacids that contain magnesium, aluminum, or calcium. Theophylline is another agent to avoid, because concurrent ciprofloxacin will cause increases in theophylline levels and possible theophylline toxicity.

Board Testing Point: Recognize that sucralfate and antacids may interfere with absorption of ciprofloxacin.

221. Answer: A

Answer: *Pseudomonas aeruginosa.*
This is the most common cause of acute otitis externa in patients with diabetes. Note: This guy needs admission and to be treated with intravenous antibiotics that cover *Pseudomonas* well to avoid the consequences of malignant otitis externa—osteomyelitis, meningitis, and brain abscess. Choices would include piperacillin/tazobactam or cefepime. The other organisms can cause otitis externa but are less common, especially in diabetics.

Board Testing Point: Know that *Pseudomonas aeruginosa* is the most likely etiology of acute otitis externa in a diabetic patient.

222. Answer: D

Answer: *Vibrio vulnificus.*
This is a classic case: an alcoholic man with liver disease who has exposure to salt water or fish and comes in with sepsis, confusion, and bullous skin lesions. Another case is a person with liver disease who eats oysters or goes to the beach. The other choices are less likely, particularly malaria and leptospirosis. Group A *Streptococcus* or a *Staphylococcus* could do this, but his history is too classic to pick anything else but *V. vulninficus* for this unfortunate man.

Board Testing Point: Recognize the association of *Vibrio vulnificus* sepsis in patients with underlying liver disease and exposure to raw fish or sea water.

223. Answer: C

Answer: Penicillin G, 3 million units intravenously q 4 hours.
This patient has neurosyphilis. But, the CSF VDRL was negative. How can he have neurosyphilis? Remember that the CSF VDRL is very **specific** (meaning that if it is positive, it means they truly have neurosyphilis), but it is not very **sensitive** (only about 1/2 of patients with documented neurosyphilis will have a positive CSF VDRL!). The serum VDRL and FTA-ABS were both positive. If you do an LP on someone with neurologic disease and they have a positive RPR or VDRL on their serum that is relatively high, then you are going to have to consider that they might have neurosyphilis. He has meningitis by definition with 50 WBCs in his CSF, and he has an elevated abnormal protein in the CSF. Both go along with neurosyphilis. And, he also has AIDS, which he didn't know he had before coming to see you.

Note: Always look for syphilis in a young person with hearing loss or in an adolescent with alopecia!

Board Testing Point: Know that with clinical signs and symptoms of syphilis and laboratory (serum VDRL and FTA-ABS) confirming syphilis in a patient with meningitis, a negative CSF VDRL does not rule out neurosyphilis.

---

224. Answer: B

Answer: Change the catheter site; add caspofungin.
She has infection with *Candida krusei*, which is almost always resistant to fluconazole and has reduced susceptibility to amphotericin B. Caspofungin and the other echinocandins (micafungin, anidulafungin) have been shown to be as effective and better tolerated than amphotericin B for *Candida krusei* infections. Literature supports removal and replacement of a central venous catheter if catheter tip cultures are positive for a *Candida* species or other fungi. **Never, never, never** consider a *Candida* blood culture result as a contaminant. Remember: With disseminated *Candida*, you do want to look for endophthalmitis and liver and splenic lesions, which she did not have at this time. Note that sometimes the liver/spleen lesions may not occur until after the neutropenia has resolved!

Board Testing Point: Recognize that *Candida krusei* is likely to be resistant to fluconazole and that an echinocandin is the best therapy for this infection.

---

225. Answer: D

Answer: *Pseudomonas aeruginosa*.
Note: He is only 5 days out from his transplant. The most common organisms to cause problems this early are hospital-acquired infections, particularly with gram-negatives like *Pseudomonas* or gram-positives like *Staphylococcus aureus*. CMV and *Pneumocystis* are likely 1–4 months out. *Cryptococcus* is a problem more often 4 or more months out. *Legionella* doesn't have much more increased incidence, unless there were something wrong with the processing of water in the hospital.

Board Testing Point: Understand which infections are most likely post-transplant based on the time frame since the transplant occurred.

---

226. Answer: C

Answer: Pyrazinamide (PZA).
Note that hyperuricemia is common but gout is rare. PZA along with INH and rifampin may cause hepatitis also. INH can cause peripheral neuropathy. Rash is seen with PZA and ethambutol; and with ethambutol, the thing to look out for is optic neuritis, particularly manifested by changes in vision, especially with colors. This is rare if the dose of 15 mg/dk/d is used.

Board Testing Point: Be familiar with the side-effect profile of the anti-tuberculous medications.

---

227. Answer: B

Answer: *Bartonella henselae*.
This patient has cat scratch fever or disease. Note: Commonly you'll see patients present with axillary nodes and scratches on the hand. But know that a classic conjunctivitis pre-auricular node syndrome is cat scratch disease. *Bartonella* is one of the few organisms other than TB that causes necrotizing granulomas. Lyme disease does not cause conjunctivitis. Herpes causes keratitis, not conjunctivitis. MRSA would cause a purulent conjunctivitis. The poor turtle here is innocent, so *Aeromonas* is not a problem either. *Aeromonas* typically would cause an exudative diarrhea. What causes lymph node swelling in a person who works with animals that does not respond to anti-staph drugs? Most common thing is going to be cat scratch.

Board Testing Point: Know that *Bartonella henselae* is responsible for cat scratch disease/fever.

---

228. Answer: C

Answer: Cytomegalovirus retinitis.
CMV retinitis is the most common eye disorder to occur in patients with CD4 counts below 50. Patients will frequently initially complain of floaters, and they will gradually lose vision. This patient has classic findings on ophthalmologic examination: attenuation of vessels in the area affected by retinitis. Retinal lesions will occur as 2 possible presentations. In the posterior type, large areas of thick white infiltrate are accompanied by retinal hemorrhage, with a distribution along retinal vessels. The peripheral type demonstrates granular retinitis with satellite lesions and less hemorrhage. Behind the advancing border is necrotic retina. Treatment is with oral valganciclovir unless she has sight-threatening lesions; then intravitreal injection/implant ganciclovir or IV ganciclovir is generally used. Also, it is important to get her HIV under better control and, with better anti-HIV therapy, raise her CD4. This would be very helpful in controlling her disease.

Board Testing Point: Recognize that in a patient with AIDS and a low CD4 count who has new onset of floaters, CMV retinitis is most likely and must be addressed quickly.

---

229. Answer: A

Answer: Staphylococcal species.
The microbiology of prosthetic valve endocarditis is related to how soon after the surgery endocarditis occurs. Early endocarditis occurs within 2 months of valve implantation and late endocarditis is after 2 months. The pathogenesis of early prosthetic valve endocarditis is that organisms are implanted at the time of surgery and thus are usually skin flora, which is why staphylococcal species predominate. The prevalence of *Staphyloccoccus aureus* vs. coagulase-negative staph is approximately the same.

Late endocarditis occurs due to bacteremias unrelated to the valve implantation surgery itself and thus resembles native valve endocarditis, with viridans streptococci being the most common infecting organism. In 2009, the International Collaborative Endocarditis published the largest review to date on prosthetic valve endocarditis. S. aureus was the cause in 23%, followed by coagulase-negative staphylococci.

Board Testing Point: Know that staphylococci are the most common cause of early prosthetic valve endocarditis.

---

230. Answer: D

Answer: Assay for acute and convalescent titers.
This patient has tularemia. To diagnose tularemia, which is due to *Francisella tularensis,* you usually will do acute and convalescent serum titers. You do **not** want to biopsy or aspirate a lymph node with tularemia. You are putting yourself and the lab at risk for aerosolization of the organism. Febrile agglutinins are **worthless**. Treatment of this man would be with IM streptomycin, IV gentamicin, or oral doxycycline. He doesn't appear to be that ill, so oral doxycycline might be worth a trial. There is a higher risk of relapse with oral doxycycline, though.

Board Testing Point: Recognize the clinical features of tularemia.

231. Answer: B

Answer: Ehrlichiosis.
This patient has fever and nonspecific symptoms. He has splenomegaly. He has pancytopenia with elevated liver transaminases and has visited an endemic area, Missouri. This clinical picture goes with ehrlichiosis. For tularemia, you would expect lymphadenopathy and not expect to find a pancytopenia. *Histoplasma* and *Blastomyces* would usually present with pneumonia and/or skin lesions. Missouri is not endemic for Lyme disease, and he lacks the most common presenting symptom of Lyme disease—erythema migrans.

Board Testing Point: Recognize the clinical features of ehrlichiosis.

232. Answer: A

Answer: *Neisseria gonorrhoeae.*
She has the classic findings of disseminated gonococcal infection (DGI). Two main syndromes of DGI are 1) polyarthralgia/dermatitis/tenosynovitis (as in this case), and 2) purulent arthritis without skin lesions. Overlap syndromes may also occur.

Note: If she was having menses, or recently completed her menstrual period, that would have been even more indicative of this type of infection. Other risk factors include pregnancy and SLE. Remember that women are more likely than men to have this infection. It is unlikely that you will grow the organism from the blood, but possibly from the genitourinary tract. However, concurrent symptomatic genital infection is rare. The other thing to remember is that ceftriaxone is the treatment of choice because of the resistance problem with penicillin and the quinolones in the United States. None of the other choices would fit this picture except for possibly *Streptococcus pyogenes*—but endocarditis would have to be in the differential, and she has no evidence of this from the history.

Board Testing Point: Recognize the clinical features of disseminated *Neisseria gonorrhoeae* in a sexually active person.

233. Answer: D

Answer: *Mycobacterium tuberculosis.*
This man most likely has AIDS. He has scattered lymphadenopathy with lower lobe infiltrates. He does not have severe hypoxia or disseminated diffuse disease on CXR, helping to differentiate TB from *Pneumocystis*. The hilar adenopathy helps you lean toward tuberculosis also. The other organisms are much less likely. Look for *Bartonella* with skin lesions; *Rhodococcus* is possible but much rarer than *Mycobacterium tuberculosis*. He has no travel history to suggest that coccidioidomycosis should be considered.

Board Testing Point: Recognize that tuberculosis is very likely in the HIV-infected population, and know its clinical presentation.

234. Answer: A

Answer: Oral fluconazole.
She has cystitis with yeast likely to be sensitive to fluconazole and more than likely due to the urethral catheter that should have been removed days ago. Fluconazole has > 90% oral bioavailability and is excreted in the urine, so it would not need to be given IV to treat cystitis. You would not subject this woman to IV amphotericin B, and oral administration works only for oral and esophageal candidiasis because it is not absorbed. Re-insertion of the indwelling urethral catheter is not a good idea, because you will likely just perpetuate her symptoms with continued colonization of her bladder.

Board Testing Point: Recognize that candidal cystitis in a diabetic patient requires therapy.

235. Answer: C

Answer: HIV ELISA.
Patients with HIV infection have an increased risk of having recurrent infections with *Salmonella*. All *Salmonella* are now considered to be in a single species, *S. enterica*, with various serotypes that were previously considered to be seperate species, such as *typhimurium*. **Know this**: If someone has recurrent bacteremias with *Salmonella enterica* or *Streptococcus pneumoniae*, think about HIV! If you have a patient from Southeast Asia who is growing *Penicillium marneffei,* then also think about HIV. The other choices are much less likely to be helpful in this patient. Be aware also that complement deficiency can predispose to these infections too, as well as sickle cell patients and others without functional spleens. I'd also be worried about endocarditis and consider an echocardiogram as well.

Board Testing Point: Be suspicious of HIV infection in a young person with recurrent bacteremias or pneumonias.

236. Answer: D

Answer: *Clostridium tetani.*
This man has **tetanus**! Look for it in elderly people who have likely not been immunized in years. Classically, they will present with "lockjaw" and then progress to have the other symptoms. The weird opisthotonic posturing described is classic for tetanus. Note: The only other thing that will do this is strychnine poisoning. Dystonic reactions to drugs can also look like this, but remember that usually this involves **lateral head turning**, which is very rare in tetanus. Dental infections may produce trismus but do not cause the other manifestations of tetanus.

Treatment is well laid out in many texts: Always protect the airway; administer diphenhydramine to be sure you are not dealing with a dystonic reaction; then proceed to giving a benzodiazepine to control spasms and decrease rigidity. Treatment consists of administering human tetanus immunoglobulin and immunization with Td (tetanus toxoid). Metronidazole is also given for 7–10 days. The course can be quite prolonged and require 6–8 weeks of intense rehabilitative therapy. Patients will receive 3 Td doses over the period of 8 weeks.

Board Testing Point: Recognize the clinical presentation for tetanus.

---

237. Answer: A

Answer: Begin combination antiretroviral therapy.
She most likely has HIV-related immune thrombocytopenia—this is very common in HIV-infected individuals. Treatment with combination therapy has shown to be most effective. The 2014 DHHS guidelines recommend using a non-nucleoside reverse transcriptase inhibitor (NNRTI): efavirenz plus tenofovir/emtricitabine or atazanavir-ritonavir plus tenofovir/emtricitabine, or a boosted protease inhibitor (PI): atazanavir/ritonavir plus tenofovir/emtricitabine or darunavir/ritonavir plus tenofovir/emtricitabine, or an integrase inhibitor (INSTI) such as raltegravir plus tenofovir/emtricitabine.

Steroids would be contraindicated in this immunocompromised patient, and we have no evidence that parvovirus B19 might be involved with a severe anemia, so use of IVIG is also not warranted. She is not actively bleeding and her platelet count is above 20,000, so there is no need to transfuse her with platelets at this time. Her CD4 count is too high to begin trimethoprim/sulfamethoxazole. Her CD4 count is < 350 cells/microL, which is the recommended cut-off for initiating antiretroviral therapy. Know that the cutoff for starting HIV medications is 350 (and also remember that for PCP prophylaxis it is < 200; MAC prophylaxis < 50).

Board Testing Point: Recognize thrombocytopenia as a common manifestation of HIV infection and that effective therapy for the HIV infection will usually help resolve the thrombocytopenia.

---

238. Answer: B

Answer: *Yersinia enterocolitica.*
Certain organisms, such as *Yersinia enterocolitica*, are iron-loving (siderophoric) and grow better in the presence of high iron concentrations. Thus, iron overload states (from frequent transfusions or hereditary hemochromatosis) promote their virulence. *Y. enterocolitica* may grow in stored, packed red cells if contaminated by an infected donor. It also can harvest iron bound to deferoxamine. It causes an inflammatory diarrhea with or without the sepsis syndrome. Other sidephoric organisms include *Listeria monocytogenes* and *Vibrio vulnificus*. The former typically causes meningitis, and the latter, necrotizing fasciitis. Although *E. coli* can cause an inflammatory diarrhea, it is not siderophoric. The other organisms listed would not cause an inflammatory diarrhea.

Board Testing Point: Recognize the association of *Yersinia enterocolitica* bacteremia with a history of sickle cell disease with multiple transfusions and deferoxamine use.

---

239. Answer: E

Answer: Continue INH; repeat serum aminotransferase measurements in 1 month or sooner if clinically warranted.
Otherwise healthy individuals with no history of liver disease should be monitored monthly for symptoms of hepatotoxicity; e.g., nausea, vomiting, right upper quadrant pain, jaundice. Routine monitoring of transaminases is not recommended, and, if performed, should not be used as a reason to discontinue INH if ≤ 5 x normal. This is because approximately 20% of patients started on INH will have such transaminase elevations with no ill consequences, and switching to another regimen unnecessarily promotes resistance and removes INH as a potent treatment of active TB if it occurs. Patients with underlyting liver disease, HIV infection, pregnancy or ≤ 3 months postpartum, drink alcohol regularly, or take other medications that have potential liver toxicity effects should have transaminases monitored monthly. Addition of pyridoxine has no effect on the hepatotoxicity of INH and is indicated only in patients at high risk of peripheral neuropathy; e.g., elderly, malnourished, alcoholic, renal failure, pregnancy, or lactating.

Board Testing Point: Recognize that up to a 5x elevation in AST and ALT are allowed in asymptomatic patients taking INH.

240. Answer: C

Answer: Both hepatitis B vaccine and hepatitis B immunoglobulin at birth.
The mother is most likely a carrier of hepatitis B infection. She will pass this to her newborn infant at delivery with 90% efficiency if there is no intervention; therefore, the child should receive both hepatitis B immuneglobulin as well as vaccine within the first 12 hours of birth! They should be given in 2 separate sites because it is more effective for any instance in which you are giving an "immunoglobulin" type product and the vaccine concurrently. Otherwise, the immunoglobulin will "bind up" the vaccine and prevent an immunologic response from occurring in the recipient of the vaccine. Note that this scenario would also work for someone who was exposed to a person with hepatitis B—as with a sexual exposure or a needlestick exposure. Note also that if the exposed person has received vaccine and is known to be immune, you don't have to do anything because that is the purpose of the vaccine—it will protect the exposed person.

Board Testing Point: Know to give an infant born to a hepatitis B surface-antigen-positive mother both hepatitis B immunoglobulin and hepatitis B vaccine at delivery.

241. Answer: C

Answer: *Mycobacterium marinum.*
Think about this organism in someone who is around water and marine organisms. For humans, the most common method of getting this is minor trauma, particularly contact with fish spines or crustaceans. Fish tank and swimming pool outbreaks have also occurred. The infection takes a while to incubate, usually 2–3 weeks, and obviously will not respond to routine antibiotics. Sporotrichosis, chromomycosis, and blastomycosis can also all present like this—but nothing in the history helps us think about these. *Vibrio vulnificus* is also associated with water, but you would expect to see **bullous** skin lesions; and it is usually seen in someone with liver disease, particularly alcoholics. *S. pyogenes*, *C. septicum*, and *S. aureus* may all cause skin and soft tissue infections in other settings. *Bartonella crustacea* does not exist.

Board Testing Point: Recognize the clinical features and risk factors for *Mycobacterium marinum* infection.

242. Answer: E

Answer: Herpes simplex virus.
Even though this man has been in an area with possible tularemia, it is very unlikely to present in this fashion. He has not been in an endemic area for Lyme disease (*Borrelia burgdorferi*). *Listeria* and *Streptococcus* are much less likely, based on his CSF findings. The protein and glucose are normal, which more likely indicates a viral etiology, although the protein is commonly elevated in herpes encephalitis. His confusion indicates encephalitis is also occurring, which more commonly occurs with herpes infection than with any of the other organisms listed. The EEG findings localized to the temporal lobe area are classic for herpes encephalitis. PCR of the CSF would be the best diagnostic test to detect herpes simplex virus. IV acyclovir is the treatment of choice.

Board Testing Point: Recognize the clinical features of herpes encephalitis and the characteristic focality of the EEG to the temporal lobe area.

243. Answer: C

Answer: Fluoroscope-guided aspiration of the hip.
You need to attempt to identify an organism before starting therapy. It is likely to be *Staphylococcus,* but it could be either sensitive or resistant to methicillin. Other organisms are possible because a previous surgery is involved. This is a chronic problem, and blood cultures are likely not to be helpful. The bone scan really is not of any help either—we know he has bone involvement by plain films. Starting therapy at this point is not prudent, and it is probable that he will need removal of the prosthesis and debridement of the area.

Board Testing Point: Recognize that diagnostic studies should be done before empirically treating an infected prosthetic hip joint.

244. Answer: A

Answer: Enterotoxigenic *Escherichia coli.*
She had traveler's diarrhea. This is usually a nonbloody diarrhea that resolves without treatment. Eating leafy vegetables or uncooked foods will expose travelers to this organism. Additionally, ice and water are common sources, especially since travelers mistakenly think that ice is protected. Also, a few people feel like the alcohol in a mixed drink will kill the bacteria—but it doesn't work that way. The other bacteria listed would generally cause much longer symptoms and more extensive disease. Remember: With *E. coli* O157:H7, do not give antibiotics because of the perceived increased risk of hemolytic-uremic syndrome. Rotavirus is unlikely, and you would expect it more often in a daycare setting or with exposure to children, and it would not be likely in a "travel" question.

Board Testing Point: Recognize the most common cause of traveler's diarrhea.

245. Answer: C

Answer: Neurocysticercosis.
This term is used for human CNS infection with *Taenia solium* cysts. Most literature involves intracerebral cysts that cause seizures and mass effects. Intraventricular cysts, as well as subarachnoid cysts, can also occur. Drug therapy with albendazole is the treatment of choice. Sometimes, corticosteroids are also required if CNS inflammation is severe or causing symptoms. He does not have HIV, so that really throws *Toxoplasma* and *Cryptococcus* out the window. Cystic lesions would be very unusual with lymphoma. HSV should not do this normally.

Also with this, think of someone with seizures who has this lesion but who hasn't traveled anywhere. The kicker is that they live with a housekeeper or someone who has the infection and is transmitting it fecally/orally in the house.

Board Testing Point: Recognize the clinical manifestations of neurocysticercosis.

---

246. Answer: D

Answer: *Staphylococcus aureus*.
What gives you hypotension with a rash and multi-organ involvement with a history of trauma? Toxic shock syndrome! And that is what this poor man has. The dog bite may have tricked you, but remember he is **not** immunocompromised. Disseminated *Pasteurella* and *Eikenella* are really unusual and unlikely to give you this constellation of findings—endocarditis, yes, but multi-organ involvement, no. *Bartonella henselae* (cat scratch fever) would not do this either. Then we have *Neisseria,* and it is possible, but the trauma history is what should have led you to *Staphylococcus*.

Board Testing Point: Recognize the clinical presentation for toxic shock syndrome and be aware of the clinical constellation as seen with this patient.

---

247. Answer: E

Answer: False-positive HIV ELISA for HIV-1.
She never should have been told she had HIV infection. False-positive HIV ELISAs are quite common; that is why we must wait for the Western blot results. Unfortunately, indeterminate Western blots are also seen occasionally. Indeterminate Western blots generally are false-positive results and are positive in only 1 band that is tested. The other thing to note is that this patient is really at low risk. When you test a low-risk population with a highly sensitive test, you are likely to see a large number of false-positive test results. It was possible early on that this was early HIV-1 infection; however, by 3 months and 6 months, she should have developed more bands. Resolved HIV infection in adults has not been clinically described. HIV-2 infection would show up on the Western blot. The other choice that this is a false-negative Western blot is very unlikely at this point. Additionally, the best test to help discern this woman's status would be an HIV viral load or an HIV PCR DNA test (qualitative). These would be useful early in determining if her indeterminate Western blot was a false-positive.

Board Testing Point: Know how to evaluate a low-risk patient with an indeterminate HIV serology test.

---

248. Answer: Answer: C

Answer: Atovaquone/proguanil (250 mg/100 mg): 1 tablet daily beginning 1 day before departure, and continuing during travel until 1 week after return.
All 4 drugs—chloroquine, mefloquine, atovaquone/proguanil, and doxycycline—are effective for chemoprophylaxis against malaria **if** dosed correctly and regional resistances are accounted for!

Chloroquine, mefloquine, and doxycycline act on blood stages of the malaria parasites following their maturation in the liver. So, they should be continued for 4 weeks after return from an endemic area.

There is widespread chloroquine-resistant malaria in West Africa. So, chloroquine should not be used for chemoprophylaxis in that area.

Atovaquone/proguanil is active against both blood and tissue stages of the parasite life cycle. So, it interferes with development of actively replicating parasites in the liver and can, therefore, be discontinued 1 week after the end of exposure.

Board Testing Point: Know malaria chemoprophylaxis for travelers.

249. Answer: C

Answer: Pap smear, RPR, HIV testing and counseling, and gonorrhea and *Chlamydia* culturing.
The patient likely is colonized; and so, even if you find the organism, it doesn't necessarily mean that it is causing the problem. You must determine if she has gonorrhea or C*hlamydia*. Both are treatable diseases. It is important for her to know and for the public health officials in the community to be aware of either of these infections so that partner notification can occur. Because of her sexually active state with multiple partners, she should be tested for HIV and syphilis, and undergo a pap smear. Additionally, if not immunized, she should receive the HPV vaccine.

Note that HSV culturing is not likely to be helpful. If she is asymptomatic, you would not treat her even if she had positive cultures, and HSV would not be causing her discharge. Culturing for *Gardnerella* is not cost-effective, is difficult to do, and likely would not yield meaningful results. *Candida* culturing is not going to be helpful.

Board Testing Point: Recognize that a sexually active teenager with symptoms should be appropriately tested and receive counseling about sexually transmitted diseases.

250. Answer: E

Answer: No prophylaxis is indicated.
The source patient's HIV viral load is really high, so we would offer him the 3-drug therapy list of zidovudine, lamivudine, and indinavir for 4 weeks. No data exists (at least as of February 2009) on whether you should change therapy based on genotypes. Some authorities currently recommend considering it. Remember: For large amounts of infectious fluid exposure with a high viral load, use 3-drug prophylaxis! For noninfectious fluid or fluid that is in contact with "intact skin only," no prophylaxis is indicated.

Note that urine is not on the list of body fluids with which to be worried about transmission. Blood, semen, vaginal secretions, CSF, synovial, pleural, peritoneal, pericardial, and amniotic fluids are considered "potentially infectious." Let's say this was blood in a cup. He would have exposure to a large volume of blood to what would be considered "skin with integrity potentially compromised."

Board Testing Point: Know that exposure to urine from an HIV-infected patient does not warrant HIV prophylaxis in the health care setting.

---

251. Answer: B

Answer: Cefotetan.
Ingestion of alcohol by patients receiving cephalosporins containing the MTT (methylthiotetrazole) moiety at position 3 has been associated with disulfiram-like reactions. The MTT group's configuration is similar to disulfiram, and appears to block alcohol metabolism at the acetaldehyde step. The accumulation of acetaldehyde is associated with these symptoms. The antibiotics with the MTT side group are cefotetan, cefamandole, cefoperazone, moxalactam, and cefmetazole (the latter 2 are no longer available in the U.S.). Note that these agents also inhibit vitamin K 2,3—epoxide reductase, which converts inactive vitamin K to its active form. Therefore, in a patient with already depleted vitamin K (like an alcoholic or someone with liver disease), use of these antibiotics could increase the PT and cause bleeding problems.

Board Testing Point: Recognize that cephalosporins that contain the MTT side group may result in disulfiram-like reactions or bleeding disorders.

---

252. Answer: E

Answer: No further infectious workup is indicated.
He has classic signs of depression, with changes in sleeping and eating patterns and loss of interest in usual entertaining activities. EBV serology has been blamed for many things, from chronic fatigue to a persistent EBV syndrome. He has a completely normal examination. You have no documentable symptoms except his fatigue, and he has had major life complications in the past year. These patients can be very difficult to convince that depression could be at the root of their problem. Frequently, it takes a combination of medication as well as an effective counselor to help these patients get back to a normal life. After starting on an antidepressant and receiving counseling, he returned to his youthful healthy self, lost 30 lbs in 6 months, and was remarried 3 years later. Not all patients are success stories like this, but it should be remembered that a nonspecific laboratory test, if misinterpreted, can frequently cause more harm than good.

Board Testing Point: Recognize that isolated laboratory tests reviewed without clinical information may yield misleading information.

---

253. Answer: A

Answer: Trimethoprim/sulfamethoxazole.
This patient with advanced HIV disease develops hyperkalemia while being treated for PCP. TMP/SMX can block tubular potassium secretion, and severe hyperkalemia has been reported in AIDS patients receiving IV TMP/SMX for the treatment of PCP. Hyperkalemia has also been reported in elderly patients receiving oral TMP/SMX. Although adrenal insufficiency can cause hyperkalemia and does occur in patients with advanced HIV disease, it would be unlikely in this patient, because he received steroids.

Board Testing Point: Recognize that trimethoprim/sulfamethoxazole can result in hyperkalemia.

254. Answer: B

Answer: No therapy at this time.
This patient is asymptomatic but has a positive urine culture for a frequently drug-resistant organism. Most chronically catheterized patients will have positive urine cultures. Treatment should occur only if the patient has a symptomatic infection. This patient is asymptomatic, including a normal WBC. Attempted treatment would likely lead to a more drug-resistant organism without offering benefit to the patient.

Board Testing Point: Recognize that asymptomatic bacteriria in a patient with an indwelling Foley catheter does not usually require antibiotic therapy.

255. Answer: C

Answer: Associated with cough.
Angiotensin-converting enzyme inhibitors are effective antihypertensive agents, with rare side effects of cough (10%), reversible renal insufficiency, hyperkalemia, and angioedema (< 0.1%). They have been proven effective in slowing the rate of progression of diabetic and other proteinuric renal diseases. Discontinuation rates for hyperkalemia are low (< 1% in studies). Patients with renal artery stenosis often have an exaggerated response to converting enzyme inhibitors. Renin levels are high in patients taking these agents.

Board Testing Point: Recognize the effects of angiotensin-converting enzyme inhibitors.

256. Answer: B

Answer: Order a transesophageal echocardiography (TEE).
This patient has a history of aortic stenosis, which increases his risk for infective endocarditis. The presence of a fever and a worsening murmur further increases the pretest probability for this disease. The presence of *S. aureus* bacteremia practically gives away the diagnosis, but confirmatory imaging can help confirm the diagnosis and plan therapy.

A TTE is a reasonable initial test because it is not invasive. However, it is less sensitive compared to a TEE. Therefore, if the TTE is negative but, as in this case, clinical suspicion remains high, the next step should be a TEE. Following a normal TTE, this patient has several indications for a TEE, including persistently positive blood cultures with an organism known to be a common cause of infective endocarditis.

Persistence of fever and bacteremia in follow-up blood cultures 2–4 days after initiation of appropriate antibiotic therapy in the absence of removable focus of infection warrants:

1) ruling out deep-seated infection, including infective endocarditis, and
2) prolonged antibiotic therapy of 4–6 weeks (thus, "continue treatment with vancomycin 2 weeks" is wrong).

Vancomycin or daptomycin is the treatment of choice. Linezolid is not recommended for treatment of *Staphylococcus aureus* bacteremia. Addition of gentamicin to the treatment of *S. aureus* bacteremia or native valve endocarditis is not recommended.

Board Testing Point: Recall the diagnostic testing and management of *Staphylococcus aureus* bacteremia. Know that TEE is indicated if TTE is negative and clinical suspicion is still high for infective endocarditis.

257. Answer: B

Answer: Metronidazole 500 mg PO tid x 10 days *or* vancomycin 125 mg PO qid 10 days.
Given the clinical presentation, the patient very likely has *Clostridium difficile*-associated diarrhea (CDAD) (severe watery diarrhea that developed when in the hospital while on antibiotics) and risk factors: age, recent antibiotic therapy with levofloxacin. The most common antibiotics that cause CDAD are the fluoroquinolones, penicillins, cephalosporins, and clindamycin.

There are various ways to determine severe vs. nonsevere disease. Typically, they include leukocytosis (WBC > 15,000–20,000), fever, significantly elevated serum creatinine, and severe abdominal pain. When the signs and symptoms are suspicious for CDAD, empiric therapy is started before toxin assay results are back.

For **non**severe CDAD, either metronidazole 500 mg PO tid x 10 days **or** vancomycin 125 mg PO qid. 10 days is appropriate treatment. But for **severe** CDAD, give vancomycin 125 mg PO qid 10 days (treatment failures with metronidazole). If the patient with severe CDAD cannot tolerate oral therapy, then intracolonic vancomycin (per enema) plus intravenous metronidazole is required.

Board Testing Point: Recognize clinical severity and appropriately manage *C. difficile*-associated diarrhea.

258. Answer: A

Answer: Despite symptom resolution, antibiotic therapy is appropriate to prevent transmission.
Shigella is a virulent pathogen and is transmitted by person-to-person contact or by ingestion of food or water contaminated with human feces. *Shigella* are acid-resistant and survive transit through the stomach. It is estimated that as few as 10–100 organisms can cause disease. *Shigella* gastroenteritis usually presents as mucoid and bloody diarrhea with abdominal cramping. It can cause several extraintestinal complications, including seizures, reactive arthritis, and hemolytic uremic syndrome.

Shigella gastroenteritis is generally self-limited, lasting about 7 days. So, antibiotic therapy is not necessary for symptom resolution although it will shorten the duration by about 2 days. But, to prevent transmission, most public health officials recommend antibiotic therapy for patients with a positive stool culture (*Shigella* are present in the diarrheal stools of infected persons while they are symptomatic and for up to a week or 2 afterwards).

Antibiotic resistance is very common in the developing world and is increasing in the U.S. Therefore, antimicrobial susceptibility testing is recommended prior to treatment (i.e., no empiric therapy). Over 40% of isolates in the U.S. are resistant to TMP/SMX. (So, that answer option is wrong on 2 counts!)

Treatment: Antibiotics as above. Hydration is indicated as needed to compensate for fluid loss. Intestinal antimotility drugs such as diphenoxylate/atropine or loperamide should be avoided.

Repeat stool cultures are of no use.

Board Testing Point: Know how to manage *Shigella* gastroenteritis.

259. Answer: A

Answer: Oral trimethoprim/sulfamethoxazole 160/800 mg (1 DS tablet) bid x 3 days.
With the absence of fever or flank pain/CVA tenderness, this patient has uncomplicated cystitis (in absence of pregnancy, voiding abnormalities, comorbidities). Specific combinations of symptoms (e.g., dysuria and frequency without vaginal discharge or irritation) raise the probability of UTI to more than 90%, effectively ruling in the diagnosis based on history alone. *E. coli* is the cause of 75% to 95% of cases of uncomplicated cystitis and pyelonephritis in women.

Obtaining a urine culture prior to initiation of therapy is warranted if symptoms are not characteristic of UTI, if symptoms persist or recur within 3 months following prior antimicrobial therapy, or if a complicated infection is suspected.

The following regimens are recommended for treatment of acute uncomplicated cystitis:

- Trimethoprim/sulfamethoxazole 160/800 mg (1 DS tablet) bid x 3 days, or
- Nitrofurantoin 100 mg bid x 5 days, or
- Fosfomycin trometamol 3 g single dose

IV ceftriaxone is an appropriate choice for complicated cystitis or pyelonephritis. Ciprofloxacin is no longer recommended because of concerns for "collateral damage" (such as selection of drug-resistant organisms). It should be reserved for important uses other than acute cystitis.

Board Testing Point: Know the treatment of acute uncomplicated cystitis.

260. Answer: C

Answer: Atovaquone/proguanil (250 mg/100 mg): 1 tablet daily beginning 1 day before departure, and continuing during travel until 1 week after return.
All 4 drugs—chloroquine, mefloquine, atovaquone/proguanil, and doxycycline—are effective for chemoprophylaxis against malaria **if** dosed correctly and regional resistances are accounted for!

Chloroquine, mefloquine, and doxycycline act on blood stages of the malaria parasites following their maturation in the liver. So, they should be continued for 4 weeks after return from an endemic area.

There is widespread chloroquine-resistant malaria in West Africa. So, chloroquine should not be used for chemoprophylaxis in that area.

Atovaquone/proguanil is active against both blood and tissue stages of the parasite life cycle. So, it interferes with development of actively replicating parasites in the liver and can, therefore, be discontinued 1 week after the end of exposure.

Board Testing Point: Know malaria chemoprophylaxis for travelers.

261. Answer: D

Answer: The patient's college dormitory roommate.
Droplet precautions (facemask if within 6 feet of patient) should be continued for 24 hours after institution of effective antibiotics in patients with suspected or confirmed *Neisseria meningitidis* infection. It is no longer necessary after 24 hours of appropriate antibiotic therapy.

Postexposure prophylaxis for *Neisseria meningitidis* infections is **not** indicated for brief exposures, as in the majority of health care workers, unless there is direct exposure to respiratory secretions (e.g., intubation, suctioning).

Prophylaxis **is** indicated for "close contacts" from 7 days prior to onset of disease to 24 hours after institution of appropriate antibiotic therapy. Close contacts generally mean within 3 feet of patient for 8 hours or in contact with respiratory secretions. These include household members, roommates, and intimate contacts. Fellow students not meeting this criteria do not need prophylaxis.

Postexposure prophylaxis regimens include: rifampin PO, ciprofloxacin PO, and ceftriaxone IM.

Board Testing Point: Know the antimicrobial postexposure prophylaxis for *Neisseria meningitidis* infections.

NEPHROLOGY

262. Answer: C

Answer: Nephrogenic diabetes insipidus.
Failure to concentrate urine (i.e., achieve a urine osmolality greater than 300–400 mOsm/L) in the face of substantial hypertonic dehydration (hypernatremia) suggests diabetes insipidus. A nephrogenic origin is suspected when there is no increase in urine osmolality after exogenous vasopressin.

Board Testing Point: Recognize the clinical characteristics of nephrogenic diabetes insipidus.

263. Answer: D

Answer: Enalapril.
Multiple studies have demonstrated reduction in proteinuria and improved renal outcomes (e.g., loss of renal function, end-stage kidney disease) with ACE inhibitors in diabetic and nondiabetic proteinuric chronic kidney disease. A renal biopsy is not usually undertaken in patients with diabetic nephropathy unless atypical features are present, which would suggest an alternative glomerular disease. Dihydropyridine calcium channel blockers are inferior to ACEIs in studies and may exacerbate proteinuria. The fractional excretion of sodium is useful in the evaluation of acute renal failure, but not chronic kidney disease, as in this case.

Board Testing Point: Recognize that ACE inhibitors are the drugs of choice for diabetic nephropathy.

264. Answer: D

Answer: Kidney stones.
Nephrolithiasis and nephrocalcinosis are a tip-off to the presence of distal RTA (Type 1 RTA). RTAs are associated with a normal anion gap metabolic acidosis. Type 4 RTA is most often associated with hyperkalemia, and diabetes is a common underlying cause. Proximal RTA (Type 2 RTA) is associated with Fanconi syndrome.

Board Testing Point: Recognize the clinical features of Type 1 (distal) RTA.

265. Answer: D

Answer: Begin therapy with recombinant human erythropoietin.
Management of anemia in these patients is important, because anemia contributes both to progression of renal disease and to cardiovascular disease. The target hemoglobin in patients with chronic kidney disease and those with end-stage renal disease is 10–11 mg/dL. Patients with values below 9 mg/dL should be started on erythropoietin therapy once iron deficiency has been excluded.

"Discontinue lisinopril" is incorrect. Both ACE inhibitors and angiotensin II receptor blockers are cornerstones in the treatment of hypertension in patients with diabetic nephropathy and help delay the progression of chronic kidney disease.

"Refer for hemodialysis" is incorrect. There are no indications to initiate dialysis in this patient. The classic manifestation of uremia begins with malaise, loss of appetite, weight loss, and progresses to nausea, vomiting, and eventual encephalopathy. Refractory hyperkalemia and volume overload are indications for dialysis initiation, but are not usually seen until the eGFR is less than 10 mL/min.

"Refer for renal biopsy" is incorrect. The diagnosis of diabetic nephropathy is almost always established on the basis of a compatible clinical and laboratory profile alone. Long-standing diabetes associated with retinopathy, nephropathy, hypertension, and even neuropathy—in the absence of another obvious cause—is adequate to make a clinical diagnosis, and therefore no biopsy is necessary. In contrast, additional workup, including a biopsy, may be warranted in patients with a very recent diagnosis of diabetes who do not have retinopathy or who have a "nephritic" urinalysis.

"Administer a nonsteroidal antiinflammatory drug" is incorrect. NSAIDs should therefore not be administered in patients with nephrotic syndrome because they worsen renal function, peripheral edema, and heart failure.

Board Testing Point: Know the appropriate use of erythropoietin in chronic kidney disease.

266. Answer: E

Answer: Administer calcium gluconate.
This patient has acute renal failure secondary to rhabdomyolysis and has developed a bradyarrhythmia secondary to hyperkalemia. The clinical presentation and the markedly elevated CPK are adequate to establish the diagnosis even before the urine myoglobin is available. It is important to realize that this test may be negative depending on when it is obtained. The presence of 4+ blood without red blood cells associated with granular casts on microscopic examination is characteristic of ATN associated with rhabdomyolysis. In patients who become oliguric, particularly with severe muscle injury, hyperkalemia can be a potentially lethal complication. Initially, T waves may become peaked, but, as hyperkalemia worsens, patients may develop variable degrees of heart block, eventually resulting in 3rd degree heart block and severe conduction delays. Such patients are at risk of cardiac arrest. The 1st step in the emergency treatment of hyperkalemia is to administer calcium to stabilize the cardiac membranes. This can be administered as 10 mL of 10% calcium gluconate over 2 to 3 minutes (with constant cardiac monitoring), followed by glucose and insulin, which will then push potassium back into the cells until the total potassium burden can be removed through dialysis or other therapy.

It is incorrect to administer sodium polystyrene sulfonate (SPS) enemas. This is inappropriate for the emergency therapy of hyperkalemia. The onset of action is several hours, and SPS should be used only in life-threatening hyperkalemia after treatment with calcium, glucose, and insulin or other agents have been administered, particularly if dialysis is not available.

Initiating dialysis therapy is not correct. Hyperkalemia and acute renal failure are clearly an indication for dialysis; however, medical therapy should always be the initial therapy while awaiting dialysis, and in patients with ECG changes, calcium should be administered. It would be appropriate to obtain urgent renal consultation in such a patient, but it would be incumbent on the treating physicians to manage the patient medically until dialysis could be initiated.

Temporary pacemaker placement is not indicated. Recognition of this patient's heart block as being due to hyperkalemia is essential in the appropriate management. In the setting of rhabdomyolysis and acute renal failure, the diagnosis of hyperkalemia as the cause of heart block must be considered, and therefore the heart block will resolve once hyperkalemia is appropriately treated. Even in patients who demonstrate hemodynamic instability, immediate treatment of hyperkalemia typically resolves heart block, and therefore pacing is usually not necessary.

To perform fasciotomies is incorrect. While fasciotomy may be necessary in patients with compartment syndromes and persistent rhabdomyolysis, this would not be appropriate initial therapy with life-threatening arrhythmia secondary to hyperkalemia.

Board Testing Point: Recognize the appropriate therapy for hyperkalemia in the face of severe ECG abnormalities.

---

267. Answer: C

Answer: The dose of lisinopril should be increased to reduce proteinuria.
Mainstays of therapy for patients with proteinuria are lowering of blood pressure to < 130/85 and the use of an angiotensin-converting enzyme inhibitor (ACEI). Prednisone is the primary therapy for FSGS. While some patients may respond quickly, other patients should be treated for 6 months before they can be declared non-responders. As with any patient with proteinuria, an ACEI (or angiotensin-receptor blocker) should be given and the dose increased to the maximum amount necessary to get a reduction in proteinuria. A recent study in patients with diabetic nephropathy who received dual ACEI and ARB showed an increased risk of hyperkalemia and acute kidney injury with no reduction in mortality, and therefore combining ACIEs and ARBs is not recommended. It is not unusual to see a small decrease in the GFR when an ACEI is given to patients with underlying kidney disease, and a small unsustained rise is not an indication to discontinue therapy. There is no evidence that patients with nephrotic syndrome are at increased risk for hyperkalemia. More often, there is activation of the renin-angiotensin system resulting in mild hypokalemic metabolic alkalosis.

Board Testing Point: Recognize the effects of angiotensin-converting enzyme inhibitors.

---

268. Answer: B

Answer: Her total body sodium is approximately normal.
In a hyponatremic patient, low urine osmolality is seen in excessive water drinking and is seen in psychogenic (or primary) polydipsia. Treatment is supportive and, while hypertonic saline should be considered in symptomatic patients with hyponatremia, this hyponatremia will likely resolve at a rapid rate with fluid restriction alone. In fact, intravenous water (D5W) is frequently needed to avoid overly rapid correction (target rise in the serum sodium of no more than 8 mEq/L over the first 24 hours). Desmopressin can also be used in this situation to prevent overly rapid correction of hyponatremia. Rapid correction of hyponatremia can lead to the osmotic demyelination syndrome, with irreversible brain damage. Diuretic abuse will lead to a higher urine osmolality when not in use, or a higher urine sodium when in use. High ADH levels lead to a concentrated urine (high urine osmolality). While the patient's volume status is mildly expanded from water, total body sodium is regulated normally and is likely negligibly lower than normal.

Board Testing Point: Recognize the clinical and laboratory features of psychogenic polydipsia.

---

269. Answer: C

Answer: Acute tubular necrosis secondary to rhabdomyolysis.
This alcoholic patient presented with an anion gap metabolic acidosis. Important considerations in the differential diagnosis of a patient like this are ketoacidosis, ingestions with either methanol or ethylene glycol, and more common problems such as lactic acidosis due to sepsis or other complications of alcoholism. Both methanol and ethylene glycol also present with an elevated osmolar gap. Methanol is metabolized to formic acid, which can cause visual symptoms and blindness; ethylene glycol is metabolized to oxalate, which can appear as calcium oxalate crystals in the urine.

Both of these intoxications should be treated with fomepazole and may require emergency dialysis. Alcoholic ketoacidosis typically presents in alcoholics who have not been eating for several days and present with hypoglycemia and acidosis primarily due to production of beta-hydroxybuterate; therefore, serum ketones will be negative. Treatment with glucose-containing fluids rapidly corrects the hypoglycemia; however, it may cause severe hypophosphatemia, and if not recognized and replaced, the hypophosphatemia can cause rhabdomyolysis. This is what happened to this patient. In patients with acute rhabdo, particularly from traumatic or crush injuries, they should be immediatedly hydrated. If the patient is non-oliguric, the urine can be alkalinized, though its effectiveness is not completely clear. Serum ketones will eventually turn positive as beta-hydroxybuterate is converted to acetoacetate. These patients may also have ketosis secondary to starvation, which does not lead to acute kidney injury or sepsis, but that was not the clinical picture in this patient. Finally, while this patient was volume depleted, he was rapidly rehydrated with appropriate fluids and therefore acute tubular necrosis would be unlikely without severe hypotension.

Board Testing Point: Know the clinical and laboratory features of alcoholic patients who present with an anion gap metabolic acidosis, as well as the complications of alcoholic ketoacidosis, which include hypophosphatemia and rhabdomyolysis.

270. Answer: B

Answer: Type 1 renal tubular acidosis.
In ambulatory patients presenting with a non-anion gap acidosis, the major differentiation is between the presence of an RTA or GI losses through diarrhea. The presence of a positive urine anion gap, which represents impairment of excretion of ammonium, is consistent with RTA. Type 4 (distal) RTA is hyperkalemic and most likely to be associated with diabetes or sometimes obstructive uropathy. These patients present with hyperkalemia, often due to hyporeninemia and hypoaldosteronism. A urine pH > 5.4 is always seen in Type 1 (distal) RTA, which is often associated with nephrolithiasis and nephrocalcinosis, in familial forms, with bilateral sensorineural hearing loss. Abnormal growth may also be seen.

While Type 2 (proximal) RTA may have an elevated serum bicarbonate; as the disorder persists, loss of bicarbonate typically leads to a urine pH that is low when patients present. The "classic" association with Type 2 RTA is Fanconi syndrome, in which there is urinary loss of glucose, phosphorus, uric acid, and amino acids resulting in renal glycosuria and hypophosphatemia and hypouricosuria. Hyperparathyroidism can be associated with Type 1 RTA, and when present, it is associated with hypercalcemia. Sarcoidosis, also associated with hypercalcemia, can also lead to kidney stones. The best therapy in this patient would depend on a 24-hour urinalysis of calcium and citrate, but usually it will be either potassium citrate or bicarbonate therapy.

Board Testing Point: Recognize Type 1 RTA and its appropriate therapy.

271. Answer: A

Answer: Primary aldosteronism.
Alkalosis is generated when H+ is lost or bicarbonate is gained by the body or contraction of the plasma volume around a fixed amout of total body bicarbonate; i.e., loss of bicarbonate-free fluid. Less common causes of alkalosis generation are H+ shifts from the extracellular to the intracellular space. The alkalosis is then maintained by the inability of the kidneys to excrete excess bicarbonate in the urine (usually driven by aldosterone and decreased distal chloride delivery). The urinary chloride concentration is the most important lab test in the workup of metabolic acidosis. Chloride-responsive alkalosis (urine chloride < 10 mEq/L) is characterized by volume depletion; examples include vomiting, nasogastric suction, and contraction alkalsois (due to remote diuretic use).

When the urine chloride is > 10 mEq/L, causes fall into 3 main categories: 1) Hyperaldosterone state (primary, secondary, or apparent); 2) Genetic mutation with renal salt-wasting (Barrter's, Gitelman's, or Liddle's syndrome); and 3) Ongoing diuretic effect.

The presence of hypertension, hypokalemia (renal potassium loss based on high urinary potassium), and alkalosis suggest that the patient has primary aldosteronism. All the other choices can result in metabolic alkalosis with hypokalemia, but these conditions won't be associated with hypertension, and the urinary chloride will be low in these conditions.

Board Testing Point: Evaluate and diagnose causes of metabolic alkalosis.

272. Answer: D

Answer: High-dose steroids and cyclophosphamide.
This patient has a representative presentation of vasculitis with weight loss, fevers, acute glomerulonephritis, and + ANCA, likely representing microscopic polyangiitis (MPA). If upper or lower respiratory manifestation were present, with granulomatous disease on biopsy, her disease would be classified as granulomatosis with polyangiitis (GPA, formerly Wegener's). The renal biopsy is consistent with a pauci-immune necrotizing GN, typical of MPA. Treatment consists of high-dose steroids and cytotoxic drugs, usually cyclophosphamide.

Azathioprine is not effective, and steroids alone are inadequate. Bed rest and diuretics might help the blood pressure, but also are inadequate therapy. The role of ACEIs has not been studied. Plasmapheresis appears to be effective for MPA/GPA only in patients with 1) dialysis-dependent renal failure at the time of presentation, 2) concurrent ANCA and anti-GBM antibody positivity, and 3) pulmonary hemorrhage.

Board Testing Point: Recognize the clinical features of microscopic polyangiitis and its therapy.

273. Answer: C

Answer: Exacerbate hypercalcemia.
Loop diuretics inhibit the Na-K-2 Cl transporter leading to natriuresis, kaliuresis, and reduction in blood pressure. They can occasionally precipitate gout, increase urinary calcium and magnesium excretion, and can be used in the treatment of hypercalcemia in the setting of volume overload. Note that loop diuretics are no longer recommended as 1st line therapy in hypercalcemia due to the risk of causing or worsening volume depletion. Thiazide diuretics diminish urinary calcium excretion and can be used to prevent recurrent kidney stones in patients with idiopathic hypercalcuria.

Board Testing Point: Know the uses and mechanism of action of loop diuretics.

274. Answer: B

Answer: Non-anion gap metabolic acidosis.
This is a non-anion gap (or normal-anion gap) metabolic acidosis. First, calculate the anion gap = Na – (Cl + HCO_3). His is normal (6–10). Next, determine if a 2nd disorder is present using Winter's or a similar formula. In this case, the predicted CO_2 matches his measured pCO_2, so it is a simple non-anion gap metabolic acidosis. The next step would be to determine the etiology of the acidosis. To determine if the cause of bicarbonate loss is renal or gastrointestinal, calculate the urine anion gap = (Na + K) – Cl. His urinary anion gap is negative, which suggests appropriately high urinary ammonium (NH_4^+) excretion = appropriate urinary acid excretion. He likely has a GI source for his acidosis; e.g., diarrhea. Although his history suggests an ingestion, this would result in a high anion gap metabolic acidosis.

Board Testing Point: Know how to interpret blood gas and electrolytes in various metabolic scenarios.

275. Answer: D

Answer: Acute renal failure secondary to rhabdomyolysis.
This patient has alcoholic ketoacidosis (AKA) and presents with the classic constellation of findings of alcohol binging, hypoglycemia, and an anion gap metabolic acidosis. The presence of 3+ blood on the urine dipstick and absence of RBC's on microscopy are consistent with a diagnosis of rhabdomyolysis. These patients usually also have hypophosphatemia, which can contribute to rhabdomyolysis. The diagnosis of alcoholic ketoacidosis may be missed, because these patients improve quickly with glucose administration, and the ketones are initially beta-hydroxybutyrate and are not detected in the serum until they are converted to acetoacetate. Recognition of the clinical syndrome allows one to monitor and appropriately replace phosphorus early in the hospitalization, to prevent complications such as rhabdomyolysis.

Note that the answer option of acute renal failure secondary to ethylene glycol intoxication is incorrect. The most important clue to the diagnosis of either ethylene glycol or methanol intoxication is an osmolar gap greater than 10. The osmolality is calculated as (2 x sodium) + (glucose/18) + (BUN/2.8). This value will be significantly greater than the measured osmolality in patients with alcohol, methanol, or ethylene glycol ingestion. Also, in patients with ethylene glycol ingestion, calcium oxalate crystals may be present in the urine, a rather important clue on Board exams. Treatment of methanol or ethylene glycol intoxication includes fomepizole and often hemodialysis. Ethanol is a 2nd line treatment if fomepizole is not available.

For the answer of methanol intoxication, an osmolar gap is usually present along with an anion gap acidosis. These patients typically present with a fruity odor and blurred vision due to the degradation of methanol to formaldehyde and formic acid, which is toxic to the optic nerve. Treatment includes fomepizole and hemodialysis.

Isopropyl alcohol is found in antifreeze and rubbing alcohol. Typically, isopropyl alcohol ingestion results in an increase in the osmolal gap but does not cause a high anion gap metabolic acidosis.

The diagnosis of hepatorenal syndrome should be suspected in patients with cirrhosis, portal hypertension, and ascites. Patients who develop acute renal failure in this setting must be evaluated for intravascular volume depletion—frequently associated with diuretics, vomiting, or bleeding—or conversely, they may develop acute renal failure due to acute tubular necrosis, related to many of the medications they receive. The diagnosis of HRS depends on demonstrating a benign urinalysis, low urinary sodium concentration (typically < 10 mEq/L), no response to volume repletion, and exclusion of obstruction or toxic causes.

Board Testing Point: Know the clinical and laboratory features and therapy for rhabdomyolysis.

276. Answer: B

Answer: Obtain an MRI of the kidneys.
Patients with membranous glomerulopathy (MGN) may present with normotension and normal renal function and, if not severe, may be treated only with an ACEI or ARB because the patient may have a spontaneous remission. Also, patients with symptomatic nephrotic syndrome, decreased GFR, and progressive disease should be treated; initial protocols typically include both corticosteroids and cyclophoshamide. Nephrotic syndrome is associated with a hypercoagulable state because of the loss of antithrombin 3; and patients with MGN are at higher risk for the development of venous thrombosis with complications such as pulmonary embolus and renal vein thrombosis (RVT). RVT should be considered in patients who have severe nephritic syndrome, especially with MGN in whom hematuria, flank pain, or acute deterioration of renal function develops. More often, however, RVT can be chronic and patients may be asymptomatic; therefore, a high index of suspicion is necessary in predisposed patients. Diagnosis may be made noninvasive using MRI to avoid the use of contrast with CT. If acute, patients should receive thrombolytic therapy, though all patients will require chronic anticoagulation.

Especially with increased edema and new onset hematura, this patient has had a sudden deterioration of renal function, which is not the typical course for membranous glomerulopathy and therefore raises the possibility of RVT. Prednisone alone is not appropriate therapy for MGN. Successful protocols use corticosteroids with either cyclophosphamide or chlorambucil. Initial studies with both ACTH gel and rituximab are promising, but they should not be used for initial therapy.

In patients with significantly reduced GFR, angiography with either iodinated contrast or gadolinium should be avoided. This patient has had a significant reduction in GFR, and it is possible that ACE inhibition is contributing to this fall in GFR. ACE inhibiton is important in all patients with significant proteinuria and is a mainstay of therapy in this patient, but if the GFR deteriorates, it is always possible that doing so is contributing to the fall in GFR. The only way to determine if this is the case is to discontinue that agent, but in this patient there is no indication to add amlodipine. Plasmapheresis is not indicated and is used in patients with rapidly progessive nephritic syndromes.

Board Testing Point: Understand the presentation and management of membranous glomerulopathy, and recognize complications of nephrotic syndrome.

277. Answer: C

Answer: Increased production of antidiuretic hormone.
In patients with severe congestive heart failure with marked reduction of cardiac output, both the renin angiotensin aldosterone system and antidiuretic hormone are stimulated. Stimulation of ADH results in water retention. This condition also occurs in patients with severe nephrotic syndrome or cirrhosis. Fractional excretion of sodium will be low, and patients require treatment with water restriction, diuretics, and sodium restriction. While there is increased sodium reabsorption due to activation of the RAS system, this results in expansion of the extracellular fluid volume and further volume expansion with edema.

An incorrect response is renal sodium losses secondary to furosemide. Hyponatremia is related more to water retention from excess ADH than from sodium losses. Both furosemide and thiazide diuretics may cause hypovolemia, stimulating ADH and renal retention of water, which results in hyponatremia. Life-threatening hyponatremia has been reported in patients recently started on thiazide diuretics due to a reduction in the diluting capacity of the kidney and increased ADH release, associated with severely restricted Na intake.

SIADH is incorrect. Diagnosis of SIADH cannot be made in the face of heart failure, renal disease, adrenal disease, or volume depletion. Patients with SIADH are normovolemic and demonstrate a urine osmolality that is inappropriately high when compared with the serum osmolality. One clue to the diagnosis frequently is hypouricemia.

Adrenal insufficiency is incorrect also. Adrenal insufficiency should be considered in all patients who present with hyponatremia and hypovolemia with an elevated urine sodium. The lack of mineralocorticoid production results in sodium wasting by the kidney and may be associated with hyperkalemia and metabolic acidosis.

The choice of hypothyroidism is incorrect. Hypothyroidism causes water retention, and patients remain euvolemic. Urine sodium will be elevated. This diagnosis should always be considered when SIADH is also suspected.

Board Testing Point: Understand the clinical and laboratory manifestations that result from activation of the renal-angiotensin system and antidiuretic hormone in severe congestive heart failure.

---

278. Answer: B

Answer: Acute interstitial nephritis.
In hospitalized patients who develop acute kidney injury, one must always consider medications as the cause. In this patient, the administration of trimethoprim/sulfamethoxazole should raise the possibility of acute interstitial nephritis. Acute interstitial nephritis (AIN) is a hypersensitivity reaction that frequently produces eosinophilia in the serum and eosinophils in the urine; however, patients may still have AIN even in the absence of this finding. Hansel stain can be more effective in demonstrating eosinophils, though Wright stain is routinely used. A recent study published in the nephrology literature confirmed that eosinophils may be seen in a variety of renal diseases and are not at all specific for acute interstitial nephritis, so this finding must be taken into context. The most common medications that cause acute interstitial nephritis are the nonsteroidal antiinflammatory drugs and antibiotics including sulfa-based antibiotics, cephalosporins, quinolones, and penicillins.

Patients with HIV who are hospitalized must be thoroughly evaluated when they develop acute kidney injury, because the differential diagnosis is broad. Many of these patients present with volume depletion when acutely ill and have prerenal azotemia, but this would be expected to improve with hospitalization and fluid administration. An appropriate evaluation with a benign urinalysis and a $FE_{na} < 1\%$ would confirm the diagnosis. The urinalysis is key to the diagnosis of acute glomerulonephritis, and without hematuria or proteinuria, GN is unlikely. Similarly, patients with HIV may either be exposed to drugs (aminoglycosides, pentamidine) or toxins (radiocontrast) that can cause ATN. The diagnosis would be confirmed by the presence of dirty brown (granular) casts in the urinalysis and a $FE_{na} > 2\%$. All of these patients should have an ultrasound of the kidney to assure that there is no obstruction. Finally, HIV-associated nephropathy is associated with chronic kidney disease, characterized by nephrotic syndrome, large kidneys by ultrasound, and often progression to renal failure over 1–2 years. These patients should be treated with antiretroviral therapy and ACE inhibitors.

Board Testing Point: Recognize the clinical characteristics of acute interstitial nephritis.

---

279. Answer: A

Answer: PR3-ANCA is likely to be positive.
This patient has a "pulmonary-renal syndrome," and one should consider Goodpasture syndrome (aka anti-glomerular basement membrane antibody disease), lupus, and granulomatosis with polyangiitis (GPA, formerly known as Wegener's), though other causes are still possible. Whenever there is a rapidly progressive glomerulonephritis, regardless of etiology, one may see crescents in Bowman's space; however,

lupus typically is associated with the presence of IgG, IgA, and IgM on immunofluorescent staining. Linear staining with IgG in the glomerular basement membrane is characteristic of anti-GBM disease/Goodpasture's. Crescents are commonly found in patients with GPA, immunofluorescence is negative, and ANCA (usually PR3) will be positive in most patients. In a patient with features of chronic upper respiratory tract disease, pulmonary involvement, and glomerulonephritis, GPA is the most likely diagnosis, and ANCA is an important diagnostic tool.

The choice of "anti-GBM antibody is likely to be positive" is incorrect, since anti-GBM disease would have positive (linear pattern) immunoflourescent staining. The antineutrophil cytoplasmic antibody is an important diagnostic study in the evaluation of any patient with acute glomerulonephritis. MPO-ANCA (p-ANCA) is most likely to be positive in patients with microscopic polyangiitis, whereas PR3-ANCA (c-ANCA) will be positive most frequently in patients with GPA. While MPO-ANCA can be positive in many other forms of vasculitis, including systemic lupus, it will be the only serologic abnormality in patients with microscopic polyangiitis.

Based on the renal biopsy, initiating plasmapheresis is an incorrect choice. Plasmapheresis is the appropriate therapy in patients with anti-GBM antibody disease who are not dialysis-dependent at the time of presentation. Plasmapheresis is also appropriate in patients with GPA who are 1) dialysis-dependent at presentation, 2) with pulmonary hemorrhage, or 3) with combined seropositivity for both ANCA and anti-GBM antibody. For this patient, the standard therapy is corticosteroids and cyclophosphamide.

Significant eosinophilia is unlikely. Eosinophilia is an important clue in the diagnosis of Churg-Strauss syndrome, not GPA. Patients with Churg-Strauss also present with asthma.

Complement levels will not be low. In this patient, without evidence of immune-mediated glomerulonephritis, there is not likely to be complement activation, and complement levels are most likely to be normal.

Board Testing Point: Recognize the clinical and laboratory findings of granulomatosis with polyangiitis.

---

280. Answer: D

Answer: This patient is not likely to develop progressive renal failure.
The most likely diagnosis in the acute onset of severe nephrotic syndrome, particularly in a younger patient, is minimal change disease, which accounts for 10–15% of nephrotic syndrome in adults. The diagnosis is confirmed by renal biopsy and, in adults, the initial treatment is corticosteroid therapy. Most patients will respond to treatment with prednisone alone, though in adults (as compared to pediatric minimal change disease), it is possible that cytotoxic therapy may need to be added later to achieve remission. Patients who relapse after prednisone therapy should be retreated, but frequent relapsers may also require cytotoxic therapy. In contrast to other types of glomerular disease, minimal change disease does not usually lead to end-stage kidney disease, although frequent relapsers can develop morbidity from long-term steroid use.

It is incorrect to choose treatment that is initiated with steroids and cytotoxic therapy to prevent progressive renal disease. Initial therapy of adult minimal change disease is with prednisone alone, with cytotoxic therapy being added only for patients who frequently relapse or in whom remission cannot be achieved.

A less likely diagnosis is focal and segmental glomerulosclerosis (FSGS). Focal and segmental glomerulosclerosis is an important cause of idiopathic nephrotic syndrome in adults and is the most common cause in African-Americans. Particularly in young African-American adults, presentation with idiopathic nephrotic syndrome, hypertension, and progressive renal failure strongly suggests the diagnosis of FSGS. FSGS is also treated with prednisone initially but has a lower likelihood of response than minimal change disease, with a much higher likelihood of progression to end-stage kidney disease.

Another incorrect choice would be treatment initiated with cyclosporine. While cyclosporine has been used for treatment of steroid-resistant minimal change disease in children, it is not considered initial therapy in either adults or children. It has been used in some trials in both steroid-resistant minimal change disease and steroid-resistant focal segmental glomerulosclerosis with variable degrees of success.

Finally, ACE inhibitor therapy should be used in patients with heavy proteinuria. ACE inhibitors exert an important antiproteinuric effect and should be used in patients with hypertension and proteinuria. However, they may also be an important adjunct to therapy in patients with heavy proteinuria even with normotension.

Board Testing Point: Recognize the clinical features of minimal change disease.

281. Answer: C

Answer: Order complement levels.
This patient has isolated microscopic hematuria. The presence of RBC casts establishes the diagnosis of glomerulonephritis; therefore, complete serologic studies to exclude secondary causes are essential. The most likely diagnosis in a patient with gross hematuria immediately following an upper respiratory infection is IgA nephropathy. While the diagnosis can be established only by renal biopsy, it is not urgent since his renal function is stable and he is asymptomatic aside from the gross hematuria. It is appropriate to first check complement levels to exclude underlying secondary causes such as lupus, postinfectious glomerulonephritis, or HCV-associated GN.

Referral to urologist is incorrect. It is essential to determine in patients with hematuria whether the bleeding is most likely coming from the upper or lower tract. Clues to the diagnosis of upper tract bleeding include the presence of red blood cell casts, proteinuria associated with hematuria, and dysmorphic red blood cells. In patients with isolated hematuria where none of these features are present, urologic evaluation would be appropriate, particularly in older patients where the diagnosis of GU malignancy must be excluded. This patient has glomerulonephritis, based on the RBC casts, and urologic referral would only delay diagnosis.

Immediate referral for renal biopsy is incorrect. Patients who present with evidence of glomerulonephritis will usually require renal biopsy to establish a diagnosis. Of particular concern are those patients with acute glomerulonephritis, as manifested by evidence of salt and water retention with renal insufficiency. Patients with rapidly progressive glomerulonephritis, in which renal function can deteriorate even on a daily basis, should always be evaluated for urgent renal biopsy to quickly establish a diagnosis and initiate appropriate therapy. In this patient, outpatient evaluation should be performed before biopsy is performed.

It is incorrect to begin prednisone 60 mg daily. Patients with IgA nephropathy and normal renal function, especially without proteinuria, require no therapy. Of greater concern are patients with significant proteinuria (> 1 g/day) who are more likely to have progressive loss of renal function. More recent studies have evaluated the use of both steroid and cytotoxic therapy in patients with proteinuria and progressive renal disease in IgA nephropathy, with data suggesting these treatments may be of benefit. This would not be appropriate in this patient, as he appears to have minimal proteinuria.

Hearing evaluation is not indicated. One of the considerations in younger patients who present with hematuria due to glomerulonephritis is Alport syndrome (hereditary nephritis). The hallmarks of this disorder are hearing loss and glomerulonephritis, occasionally with associated ocular abnormalities. This disease is typically expressed much more severely in men than in women. While the family history can be very suggestive, the diagnosis can be established with certainty only by renal biopsy demonstrating particular thinning or lamellation of the glomerular basement membrane, seen on electron microscopy.

Board Testing Point: Recognize the value of checking complement levels as the 1st test in a patient with glomerulonephritis and hematuria.

282. Answer: C

Answer: Metabolic acidosis, respiratory alkalosis, metabolic alkalosis.
While it is apparent that this patient has diabetic ketoacidosis, it may not be apparent that she has a triple acid-base disorder. In evaluating all patients with electrolyte and acid-base disorders, the anion gap must be calculated. In this patient, the anion gap is 26 (high!), which is consistent with diabetic ketoacidosis. Next, calculate what the pCO_2 should be for a patient with a metabolic acidosis and a serum bicarbonate of 18. The PCO_2 should be $(1.5 \times HCO_3 + 8) +/- 2 = 35 +/- 2$. This patient's PCO_2 is 20; therefore, she is overventilating and has a superimposed respiratory alkalosis. The "delta anion gap," or change in the AG from normal, is (actual AG–normal AG) = (26–10) = 16. In a pure HAGMA, the fall in bicarb should be about the same as the rise in AG. This patient's fall in bicarb is 24 – 18 = 6. Since the fall in the bicarb is less than the increase in the anion gap, there must be a concomitant metabolic alkalosis (i.e., source of excess HCO_3) in addition to the anion gap metabolic acidosis. In this case, the metabolic alkalosis is due to gastric H+ loss (equivalent to HCO_3 gain) from severe vomiting. Appropriate therapy is still fluid resuscitation and insulin administration, while watching for the development of hypokalemia.

Board Testing Point: Know how to identify and work up acid-base disorders.

283. Answer: E

Answer: Bartter syndrome.
This patient is presenting with hypokalemia and metabolic alkalosis. The differential diagnosis of metabolic alkalosis can be approached from the perspective of causes that are chloride sensitive; e.g., those with a low urine chloride: volume depletion, previous diuretic use, vomiting, post-hypercapnic alkalosis; and those with a high urine chloride: excess endogenous or exogenous steroids and surreptious diuretic use. Therefore it is extremely helpful to order urine chloride. In this case, that is not available, and there is no obvious cause of a chloride sensitive metabolic alkalosis. This patient therefore falls under the group of disorders that are associated with normotension and hypokalemic metabolic alkalosis. The major diagnostic possibilities are Bartter syndrome, Gitelman syndrome, and a patient who is surreptitiously taking diuretics.

Bartter syndrome is caused by a mutation of the Na-K 2-chloride transporter in the thick ascending limb of Henle. Bartter's is a familial disorder characterized by metabolic alkalosis, normotension, normokalemia, hypomagnesemia, and elevated renin and aldosterone levels. One way to remember this syndrome is that the patient "looks like" someone taking furosemide, and this is the only plausible option provided. Gitelman syndrome might present in a similar fashion, but the abnormality is a defect in the Na-Cl co-transporter in the distal tubule, and the patient "looks like" someone taking hydrochlorothiazide. Gitelman's may also cause hypomagnesemia, but it also causes hypocalciuria, an important differentiating feature from Bartter's. To exclude surreptitious diuretic use, one would have to obtain a specific drug screen.

Liddle syndrome is incorrect. This familial disorder is characterized by hypertension, hypokalemia, and low renin and aldosterone. It is caused by a defect in the collecting duct sodium channel. Amiloride is the appropriate treatment.

Primary hyperaldosteronism is incorrect. These patients present with hypertension, hypokalemia, and metabolic alkalosis. Renin levels are low, while aldosterone levels are high and non-suppressible. Primary hyperaldosteronism is due to either unilateral adrenal adenoma or bilateral adrenal hyperplasia.

Addison disease is incorrect. Patients with Addison disease have mineralocorticoid deficiency and therefore are normotensive or hypotensive with hyperkalemia and a metabolic acidosis.

Renal artery stenosis is incorrect. Patients with renal artery stenosis may be hypokalemic with a metabolic alkalosis, but they are hypertensive. These patients have secondary hyperaldosteronism, and therefore renin levels are also elevated.

Board Testing Point: Describe the causes of metabolic alkalosis, and distinguish between those associated with hypertension and normotension.

---

284. Answer: D

Answer: Measure parathyroid hormone level.
This patient has Stage III chronic kidney disease secondary to diabetic nephropathy. This is a clinical diagnosis established by the presence of proteinuric kidney disease associated with retinopathy and neuropathy in a long-standing diabetic. Key features in management include BP control to < 130/80 with an ACEI or ARB; therefore, one would not want to stop her lisinopril. In patients with Stage III CKD (GFR 30–59 mL/min), one must evaluate and manage anemia and metabolic bone disease. This means consider assuring that patients have adequate iron stores and deciding when/if to start an erythropoietin-stimulating agent (ESA). One does not need to measure erythropoietin levels. An ESA should be initiated only if patients are symptomatic and not based on a specific hemoglobin.

Vitamin D (25-hydroxy) and parathyroid hormone levels should be measured despite normal calcium and phosphorus levels. Elevation of hyperparathyroid levels is common, but guidelines exist as to when this elevation is excessive. Control of hyperphosphatemia by diet and phopshate binders is essential, and patients with secondary hyperparathyroidism should be treated with 25-hydroxy vitamin D if deficient and 1,25 dihydroxyvitamin D if PTH remains elevated. Dialysis is usually not indicated until the GFR is < 15 mL/min though patients should be prepared for dialysis therapy long before they reach this threshold.

Board Testing Point: List the key elements in the evaluation and management of complications of Stage III chronic kidney disease.

---

285. Answer: B

Answer: Type 1 distal RTA.
This patient has a non-anion gap (NAG) metabolic acidosis. The initial approach in NAG metabolic acidosis is to measure the urinary anion gap. This serves as a measure of urinary acidification. Normally, the urine anion gap (Urine Na + K – Cl) is negative. However, in patients with urinary acidification defects, this value will be positive. Normally, one should be able to acidify the urine in the face of metabolic acidosis. In this patient, the urine pH is 7 because he cannot secrete H+ ions across the concentration gradient in the distal tubule. These patients cannot lower their urine pH below 6.0, regardless of degree of acidosis. These patients also have hypercalciuria, and may develop nephrolithiasis and nephrocalcinosis. Congenital familial RTA is associated with hearing loss, while acquired Type 1 RTA is seen with several underlying disorders, including hyperparathyroidism and hypergammaglobulinemia. Treatment includes bicarbonate and potassium administration.

Type 2 RTA is incorrect. These patients typically "waste" bicarbonate, and therefore the urine pH is also high initially, along with a NAG metabolic acidosis. Eventually patients have no more HCO_3 to waste, and the urine pH becomes more acid. Proximal RTA may also be associated with Fanconi syndrome and urinary loss of glucose, phosphorus, uric acid, and amino acids. This disorder is not associated with nephrolithiasis or hearing loss. Important causes of acquired Type 2 RTA include multiple myeloma and heavy metals. These patients may require large amounts of bicarbonate administration to correct the acidosis.

Type 4 RTA is incorrect. Type 4 RTA is a hyperkalemic distal RTA, most commonly occurring in diabetics, but is also associated with obstructive uropathy and other forms of tubulointerstitial renal disease. It is most often caused by aldosterone deficiency. Treatment includes sodium bicarbonate administration, fludrocortisone, and/or furosemide.

Chronic diarrhea is not a correct choice. Chronic diarrhea and HCO_3 loss may cause a NAG metabolic acidosis. However, urinary acidification is normal; therefore, the urinary anion gap will be negative.

Salicylate intoxication is not likely. Salicylate intoxication causes an anion gap metabolic acidosis and is not associated with hypokalemia. Patients typically also have a respiratory alkalosis, which serves as another clue to the diagnosis.

Board Testing Point: Recognize the clinical features of Type 1 (distal) RTA.

286. Answer: E

Answer: Impaired renal excretion due to Type 4 renal tubular acidosis due to obstructive uropathy. Diabetes is the most common cause of the "classic" presentation of Type 4 renal tubular acidosis in a patient with Type 2 DM, mild chronic kidney disease and hyperkalemia. The degree of hyperkalemia can be mild; however, if these patients are treated with antihypertensives that further block the renin-angiotensin system (ACEI and ARBs) or NSAIDs, then severe hyperkalemia can be precipitated. This patient, based on his previous labs, did not have these features. However, he did have urinary symptoms consistent with chronic and now acute urinary tract obstruction—another common cause of Type 4 renal tubular acidosis. Generalized weakness, similar to that seen in severe hypokalemia, also occurs with severe hyperkalemia, as do the ECG findings seen in this patient. Obstructive uropathy can cause severe hyperkalemia and may be suspected when there are clinical signs and symptoms as well as hyperkalemia that occassionally is out of proportion to the degree of renal failure. This patient, given his ECG findings, should be acutely treated with calcium, insulin, and glucose; sodium bicarbonate could be administered as well. Foley catheter placement and renal ultrasound are necessary for acute management as well.

Acidosis can cause movement of potassium out of cells, usually in the setting of metabolic acidosis, but he has a minimal reduction in his serum bicarbonate, so his hyperkalemia is out of proportion to his degree of acidemia. Pseudohyperkalemia is unlikely in view of the ECG findings, and excessive dietary potassium intake is an extraordinarily rare cause of hyperkalemia. Finally, based on his previous labs, he has acute kidney injury, not chronic kidney disease.

Board Testing Point: Recognize the clinical characteristics of Type 4 (proximal) renal tubular acidosis. Recognize and manage acute findings of hyperkalemia.

287. Answer: E

Answer: Begin hydrochlorothiazide 25 mg/day.
This patient most likely has congenital nephrogenic diabetes insipidus. He has thirst and polyuria. His serum sodium is borderline, elevated with a relatively low urine osmolality. Neither serum nor urine suggests diabetes mellitus as a cause of his polyuria. He had a childhood history of enuresis and has never presented for medical attention. In addition, he had no response to the administration of ADH (vasopressin). Most patients with nephrogenic diabetes insipidus learn to live with their polyuria and do not consider themselves "ill." The only treatment for nephrogenic diabetes insipidus of unknown etiology is hydrochlorothiazide, since thiazide diuretics enhance distal tubule water resorption. The lifelong history of polyuria and the ability to concentrate the urine to near 300 mOsm/kg suggests that he does not have central diabetes insipidus, so neither vasopressin tannate in oil (as administered) nor desmopressin would be effective. Water restriction would result in further hypernatremia. Although it may stimulate his kidneys to concentrate his urine somewhat more than they presently do, it would not be adequate to maintain a reasonable serum osmolality. Chlorpropamide is effective in patients with partial DI since it can stimulate ADH production, but this patient does not have central DI. The patient's relative hypernatremia also argues strongly against a diagnosis of psychogenic polydipsia.

Board Testing Point: Recognize the treatment of congenital nephrogenic diabetes insipidus.

288. Answer: A

Answer: The urine test strip detects only negatively charged proteins like albumin.
Immunoglobulins (e.g., Bence-Jones proteins), which are likely what he is excreting, are positively charged and therefore are not picked up on the dipstick.

Board Testing Point: Recognize that urine dipsticks detect only proteins like albumin and do not detect many other proteins.

289. Answer: D

Answer: Na 136, K 4.8, Cl 100, HCO_3 10, Serum Creatinine 3.5, Arterial pH 7.25.
Ethylene glycol ingestion causes acute renal failure and leads to rapid accumulation of metabolic acids. Acidosis is proportionate to the degree of renal insufficiency and is characterized by a **high** anion gap (here, AG = 26). All of the other choices have a normal anion gap.

Board Testing Point: Recognize the association of ethylene glycol ingestion with a high anion gap metabolic acidosis.

290. Answer: B

Answer: Na 140, K 2.6, Cl 115, HCO_3 13, Serum Creatinine 3.5, Arterial pH 7.31, Urine pH 6.2.
Amphotericin B causes renal insufficiency with a distal tubular injury. There is a non-anion gap metabolic acidosis that is due to a distal tubular acidification defect (Type 1 RTA), with inablity to lower the urine pH. B is the only choice with a normal anion gap and metabolic acidosis.

Board Testing Point: Recognize the laboratory manifestations of amphotericin B and its renal tubular acidosis effect.

291. Answer: A

Answer: Na 136, K 5.0, Cl 102, HCO_3 20, Serum Creatinine 3.5, Arterial pH 7.36, Urine pH 5.0.
With a moderate glomerulonephritis, metabolic acidosis is usually mild, and the anion gap is only slightly elevated, if at all.

Board Testing Point: Recognize the laboratory values seen in a patient whose status is post acute post-streptococcal glomerulonephritis.

292. Answer: E

Answer: Na 140, K 6.2, Cl 109, HCO_3 20, Serum Creatinine 1.5, Arterial pH 7.36, Urine pH 5.0.
This illustrates mild renal insufficiency with disproportionate hyperkalemia and hyperchloremic (non-anion gap) metabolic acidosis. One of the most common things that does this is diabetic nephropathy. Renal tubular acidosis is due to a defect in renal acidification, which is out of proportion to any reduction in GFR. Advanced renal insufficiency itself leads to a metabolic acidosis (mixed gap/non-gap), which is due to the overall decrease in kidney function.

Board Testing Point: Recognize the laboratory values associated with Type 4 renal tubular acidosis.

293. Answer: D

Answer: Na 135, K 4.5, Cl 108, HCO_3 22, Serum Creatinine 3.5, Arterial pH 7.37, Urine pH 5.0.
If you are looking at electrolytes in a patient with possible (or known) multiple myeloma, always check the anion gap. The correct answer here is illustrating a decrease in the anion gap, which is classically seen with multiple myeloma. The apparent reduction is due to a circulating paraprotein that has a positive charge.

Multiple myeloma can less commonly cause a light chain nephropathy, resulting in a proximal renal tubular acidosis (Type 2 RTA) with hypokalemia and a normal-anion gap metablic acidosis (NAGMA). Hence, it is less likely that "Na 140, K 2.6, CI 115, HCO_3 13" will occur.

Board Testing Point: Multiple myeloma does not cause a high anion gap, metabolic acidosis, or hyperkalemia.

294. Answer: C

Answer: Selective elevation of LDL cholesterol with increased atherogenesis.
The risk of myositis is increased, but not by very much. HMG-CoA reductase inhibitors work well, but should not be combined with fibric acid derivatives.

Board Testing Point: Know that the hyperlipidemia in nephrotic syndrome is usually manifested as an elevated LDL with increased atherogenesis.

295. Answer: C

Answer: Plasma aldosterone/renin ratio measurement.
This patient has significant hypertension. He does not have a strong family history or other risk factors for essential hypertension such as obesity. Evaluation of hypertension should always include an assessment to consider secondary causes of hypertension, especially in a young, otherwise healthy person. This patient's evaluation reveals a small adrenal lesion. In the context of stage II hypertension, this would warrant further investigation. Diseases that can cause secondary hypertension and an adrenal lesion include primary hyperaldosteronism, pheochromocytoma, and Cushing disease. Hyperaldosteronism is often familial and inherited in an autosomal dominant pattern. The classic findings of familial hyperaldosteronism include hypertension and hypokalemia with a positive family history. Cushing disease often presents with physical exam findings such as supraclavicular fat pad, purple striae, and proximal muscle weakness. Classic symptoms of pheochromocytoma include headache and sweating in addition to paroxysmal episodes of hypertension. Hypothyroidism can cause hypertension, but it is not associated with an adrenal lesion. There are not any other signs or symptoms of hypothyroidism in this patient. Adrenal gland biopsy would not be recommended at this point in the evaluation when less invasive testing can better characterize the lesion.

Board Testing Point: Recognize the signs and symptoms of familial hyperaldosteronism.

296. Answer: A

Answer: Measure aldosterone and plasma renin activity.
The poorly controlled blood pressure, requiring 4 antihypertensive agents along with the low potassium, suggests hyperaldosteronism. A salt suppression test should be done only after it has been documented that the aldosterone is elevated, the plasma renin activity is low, and the PRA ratio is > 20. If aldosterone levels do not suppress after administration of saline, then the next step is an adrenal CT scan. Renal angiography might be indicated if aldosterone and renin suggest renovascular disease. Dexamethasone suppression testing is used for evaluation of Cushing syndrome.

Board Testing Point: Recognize and screen for hyperaldosteronism.

ENDOCRINOLOGY

297. Answer: B

Answer: Fasting plasma glucose.
There have been numerous recommendations published on screening for diabetes. There are currently 3 validated tests: hemoglobin A1c, fasting plasma glucose, and an oral glucose tolerance test. Hemoglobin A1c testing is now widely used in screening for diabetes. However, hemoglobin A1c testing is not valid in patients with abnormal red cell turnover, such as those with hemolytic anemia, pregnancy, blood loss/transfusions, or use of erythropoietin. Since this patient is on erythropoietin, recommended screening would use either a fasting plasma glucose or an oral glucose tolerance test. This patient underwent screening by her nephrologist with equivocal results. The current recommendation for screening and diagnosis of diabetes would be to repeat the test that indicates a diagnosis of diabetes. Since her 2-hour oral glucose tolerance test was negative, it would not be recommended to repeat this time to screen for diabetes.

For this patient, the fasting plasma glucose was > 126 mg/dL, indicating possible diabetes. If the FPG remains > 126 mg/dL on repeat testing, the diagnosis of diabetes would be confirmed. Serum fructosamine has been used as a test to monitor long-term glycemic control in patients in whom an A1c measurement would be invalid, but is not validated as a screening method to diagnose diabetes

Board Testing Point: Recognize the different indications for utilizing screening tests for diabetes.

298. Answer: B

Answer: Check TSH.
This patient has signs and symptoms of hypothyroidism. The next test that should be ordered is a TSH level, which is expected to be markedly increased. The obvious evidence for hypothyroidism includes feeling tired, moving slowly, talking slowly, and dry skin. But don't overlook the galactorrhea, pituitary mass, and mildly elevated prolactin level. At first glance, this can be mistaken for a prolactinoma, but a prolactinoma of this size (macroadenoma) should be associated with prolactin levels > 200 ng/mL. A prolactin level < 100 ng/mL should always prompt you to look elsewhere—in this case, the thyroid. Some other causes of a mildly elevated prolactin that have been ruled out include pregnancy and excessive nipple stimulation. The pituitary mass in this patient is most likely not a tumor. It is a pseudotumor composed of TSH-secreting cells (thyrotrophs), which have hypertrophied in response to TRH stimulation. TRH also stimulates the secretion of prolactin; hence the elevated levels.

"Start bromocriptine" and "refer her to a neurosurgeon" are incorrect because it is important to rule out a thyrotroph pseudotumor first, prior to any therapeutic intervention. It would be inappropriate to treat with bromocriptine or surgery. "Look for an unknown non-pituitary cancer" is incorrect because the described clinical scenario does not suggest any reason to look for a non-pituitary cancer. "Recheck the prolactin in 6–12 months" is incorrect because, although rechecking the prolactin level would be appropriate at some time in the future, her hypothyroidism must be addressed first.

Board Testing Point: Recognize that hypothyroidism can present in many different ways. If a patient presents with a pituitary macroadenoma on CT scan but has inconsistent prolactin levels (here < 100 ng/mL) **and** hypothyroid symptoms, check a TSH to rule out a thyrotroph pseudotumor.

299. Answer: A

Answer: Stop bromocriptine; continue regular follow-up with an obstetrician.
This woman has a prolactin-secreting **micro**adenoma, and the likelihood of tumor growth with small tumors during pregnancy is ≤ 2%. There is no reason to switch to cabergoline, because she has already conceived. Prolactin levels increase over the course of pregnancy, as the breasts are prepared for lactation, so there is no rationale to check PRL levels during gestation or continue bromocriptine. Because so few women with microadenomas have tumor growth during pregnancy, it is not necessary to do an MRI or visual field examination unless there are clinical signs of tumor growth (headache, visual loss, etc.).

Board Testing Point: Know how to manage a microprolactinoma during pregnancy.

300. Answer: A

Answer: Start 25 µg of oral levothyroxine and proceed with surgery.
There is inadequate evidence to justify deferring scheduled surgery in patients with mild hypothyroidism (*Arch Int Med* 145:893, 1983). 400 µg of IV levothyroxine or 25 µg of T_3 would be risky therapy in an elderly lady from a cardiovascular standpoint.

Board Testing Point: Know when to operate on a patient with hypothyroidism.

301. Answer: A

Answer: Calcium 6.0 (8.5–10.5), PTH 2 (10–65), PO_4 6.0 (2.7–4.5).
This is a classic presentation of surgically induced hypoparathyroidism. The PO_4 is elevated because of the absence of PTH, and the PTH is virtually undetectable. The other options are incorrect either because the calcium is not low, the PTH is elevated, or the PO_4 is normal.

Board Testing Point: Recognize the clinical and biochemical manifestations of hypoparathyroidism.

302. Answer: D

Answer: Thyroid glands.
This is the autosomal dominant kindred of Multiple Endocrine Neoplasia (MEN) syndrome, type 2B or 3, with the characteristic combination of pheochromocytoma, medullary thyroid carcinoma, and diffuse gastrointestinal ganglioneuromatoses (as manifested grossly at the bedside by the tongue nodules). Medullary thyroid carcinoma (MTC) originates in the thyroid parafollicular C cells, those responsible for the secretion of thyrocalcitonin. It may be either sporadic or familial. Familial forms can be isolated or an expression of MEN kindred. Mutations of the RET proto-oncogene have been identified in the germline DNA of patients with familial MTC syndromes. Genetic testing can identify patients affected by MEN and familial MTC, allowing early diagnosis and possible cure. Total preventive thyroidectomy has been recommended in all carriers of RET genetic defects, even in families at risk with mutations of the 618 or 620 codon, because the penetrance of FMTC approaches 100%, and a 100% concordance between presence of the disease and gene carrier status. This procedure would therefore represent the only possibility of achieving a 100% cure in subjects affected by familial medullary thyroid carcinoma. The primary patient's pheochromocytoma is obvious and warrants careful preoperative treatment prior to surgical removal.

Board Testing Point: Recognize that severe hypertension with headache, diaphoresis, etc., may not be cardiac in origin and may be due to other etiologies, such as pheochromocytoma (in this instance).

303. Answer: D

Answer: Switch him to cabergoline.
The question states that the patient has a prolactinoma and is being treated with bromocriptine. Unfortunately, he is experiencing considerable nausea and vomiting, which are common side effects of bromocriptine; many patients are unable to tolerate it. An alternative drug, cabergoline, is available. This drug is just as effective at reducing prolactin levels and is much less likely to cause nausea and vomiting. Unfortunately, cabergoline is expensive. In some centers bromocriptine is the initial drug of choice because it is cost effective. However, cabergoline has become the drug of choice in many centers, because it has fewer side effects and is much better tolerated.

It would be inappropriate to just stop the bromocriptine without starting the cabergoline, because without a brief period of overlap, the patient would most likely experience a flare-up in his symptoms. Resection of a prolactinoma should be done only when the mass effect of a large tumor warrants it, such as seizures or an impaired field of vision. Adding prochlorperazine for nausea is not appropriate, because he hasn't tried a course of cabergoline. Finally, the addition of cabergoline to bromocriptine should not be done. These two drugs work by the same mechanism, and using them together would not lessen the severity of the nausea and vomiting and would increase any potential side effects.

Board Testing Point: Recognize that microadenomas of the pituitary require medical therapy and that usually cabergoline is better tolerated than bromocriptine. Also recognize that the common side effects of bromocriptine are nausea and vomiting.

304. Answer: D

Answer: Start cabergoline and repeat the CT/MRI in a few days.
This patient has a large prolactinoma, and the primary physician wants it to be removed. However, in the absence of visual field defects, seizures, severe headaches, and other findings, the surgery is not emergent and can probably wait a few days. In the meantime, start the patient on cabergoline. This drug may shrink the tumor enough to avoid surgery. Though it usually takes much more than a few days to show an appreciable reduction in size, the prolactinoma may nevertheless begin to shrink within a short period of time. Beginning the preoperative evaluation is justified, but it is more important to begin cabergoline. High-dose glucocorticoids might be justified if the patient presented with neurologic symptoms, but they are not needed in this case.

Board Testing Point: Recognize that prolactinomas that are **not** causing visual field defects, seizures, or severe headaches can initially be treated medically before surgical intervention.

305. Answer: E

Answer: Check serum IGF-1 and 24-hour urine cortisol.
Whenever a pituitary incidentaloma is discovered, two main questions must be answered. One, is the mass inhibiting secretion of any pituitary tumors? Two, is the tumor secreting something? Let's review the inhibiting scenario first. Many pituitary tumors do not appear to secrete anything and are called null cell tumors. With the advent of sensitive assays, it has been learned that some of these null-cell tumors actually do secrete. They may be secreting α-chains or gonadotrophins (LH or FSH), which rarely cause symptoms. After all, what man is going to complain about larger testes or a higher sperm count? However, some of these tumors get large enough that they inhibit secretion of pituitary hormones because of a mass effect. In this patient, the tumor is a microadenoma (< 10 mm) and is too small to inhibit secretion.

The other scenario is one of excess secretion. Does the pituitary tumor secrete any hormones? Remember the main 6 anterior pituitary hormones: ACTH, LH, FSH, GH, TSH, and PRL. A fishing expedition to test all hormones is not recommended. Instead, evaluate the patient for signs or symptoms that may point toward a particular excess such as galactorrhea or loss of libido (PRL); amenorrhea (LH, FSH); weight loss, hyperdefecation, tachyarrhythmia, or heat intolerance (TSH); hypertension, hypokalemia, or alkalosis (ACTH). These findings can be very subtle or even absent in the case of a new tumor or a very small one. If your evaluation does not point toward a particular hormone, then check the adrenal and thyroid axes. A screening test for the adrenal axis is a 24-hour urine for cortisol; a value < 70 μg is normal. The thyroid axis can be checked by a TSH and T_4 drawn at any time of the day.

You are cautioned to check one more hormone. A small tumor may be secreting GH. The effects of over-secretion of GH take many years to become evident, and many more years usually transpire before it is recognized. These patients develop acromegaly and its many serious complications. Though GH is pulsatile, its effect on IGF-1 is not. Measure a random IGF-1 in any patient with a pituitary incidentaloma. In this patient, the central obesity and hypertension may indicate hypercortisolism (Cushing syndrome). Order a 24-hour urine for cortisol and don't forget to check the IGF-1 level.

"Refer him to a neurosurgeon for transsphenoidal resection of the pituitary mass" is incorrect because there are no reasons to refer this patient for surgery at this time.

"Return to your clinic in a few weeks to recheck blood pressure" is incorrect because the pituitary tumor must be evaluated and his blood pressure management must be followed.

"Discharge him from your clinic on a drug to treat hypertension and encourage him to stop riding motorcycles" is incorrect because, once again, the pituitary tumor must be evaluated.

"Check an ACTH stimulation test, TSH, and a total testosterone" is incorrect because hyposecretion of ACTH, secondary hypothyroidism, and secondary hypogonadism are not suspected.

Board Testing Point: Recognize the clinical subtleties of a pituitary incidentaloma.

306. Answer: A

Answer: Tell her that everything is normal and discharge her from your clinic.
The important point to remember for this question is that an empty sella may be normal. This patient does not present any indication of pituitary dysfunction. The history of blood loss at the time of delivery may suggest Sheehan syndrome (hemorrhagic necrosis of the pituitary), but one of the most sensitive indicators of pituitary dysfunction is ovulation. This patient was able to get pregnant 6 more times; the hypothalamic-pituitary-ovarian axis must be working properly. She does not have Sheehan syndrome, but her obstetrical history offers another clue. Her 7 pregnancies have most likely caused her empty sella. With pregnancy, the pituitary enlarges and has

a greater blood flow. This produces an upward pressure on the diaphragm covering the top of the sella, which stretches and expands the diaphragm. After pregnancy, the pituitary returns to a normal size with a normal blood flow, but the diaphragm is acellular and remains stretched. With each subsequent pregnancy, the diaphragm becomes progressively more stretched. This allows the diaphragm to bulge downward and into the sella under the pressure of the CSF fluid above it. In some cases, the diaphragm has become so loose that the CSF fluid displaces the majority of the pituitary to the periphery of the sella. A CT of the head will fail to identify pituitary tissue, and the term "empty sella" will be used. In actuality, the sella is not empty, but contains CSF fluid and normal pituitary tissue that has been pushed to the periphery. The pituitary tissue can work perfectly normally in this environment.

It is inappropriate to refer her to a neurosurgeon. Pituitary exploration may disrupt the normal functioning of her existing pituitary tissue and result in the development of hypopituitarism. While there is no evidence of pituitary dysfunction, the abdominal striae may trick some people to suspect Cushing syndrome, but there is no mention of hyperglycemia, hypokalemia, or the typical body habitus. Stretch marks are a common occurrence, especially following pregnancy. The typical stretch marks associated with Cushing syndrome are broad and appear purplish from the coloration of underlying tissue.

Board Testing Point: Recognize that empty sella syndrome is common after multiple pregnancies and frequently is non-pathologic.

---

307. Answer: C

Answer: Check FT_4 and TSH.
Many things can cause an unexplained weight loss, and depression is common in older patients. However, these symptoms are also associated with hyperthyroidism. Unfortunately, older individuals do not always exhibit the adrenergic response to hyperthyroidism. The term apathetic hyperthyroidism refers to hyperthyroidism without the usual manifestations of palpitations, heat intolerance, etc. The only sign exhibited by the patient in this question is tremor and tachycardia.

Unexplained weight loss with a long history of smoking should always make you suspicious of cancer. Most physicians would order a chest x-ray. When it comes back normal, one should rethink the case. The thyroid should be evaluated before more extensive screening for cancer takes place. Depression is common, and it may be appropriate either to begin treating him or to refer him to a psychiatrist. However, do not forget that hyperthyroidism can cause depression. If the patient has hyperthyroidism and depression, it is not appropriate to treat the depression while ignoring the hyperthyroidism. Treat the hyperthyroidism and follow the depression; the depression will often resolve once the patient is euthyroid.

Board Testing Point: Know how to identify an older patient with apathetic hyperthyroidism.

---

308. Answer: D

Answer: Begin thyroxine 25 µg PO qd.
This patient has severe hypothyroidism along with poor cardiac function. Though hypothyroidism impairs cardiac function, it also decreases the demand being placed on the heart. Thus the heart is not always working as hard in hypothyroidism as it may be working in someone who is euthyroid. There is no question that her hypothyroidism needs to be addressed, but you are being asked to choose which treatment is most appropriate. Intravenous thyroxine will rapidly correct her hypothyroidism, especially with the addition of triiodothyronine, but this will also rapidly increase the demands placed on her heart. In the face of her impaired cardiac function, this sudden increased demand could easily exceed her cardiac capacity and have dire consequences. The remaining three choices are all oral thyroxine at different strengths. The most appropriate choice in this case is the 25 µg dose. This dose will not have much effect on her hypothyroidism, so it will not greatly increase her cardiac work. The dose can be steadily increased every 3–6 weeks if she tolerates it. The best course of action is to start low and go slow. This will give her heart a chance to increase its conditioning and be able to tolerate the next dose increase.

Board Testing Point: Recognize that when starting thyroid replacement therapy in a patient with coronary artery disease or an elderly patient with comorbidities, you must begin at a small dose to prevent complications.

309. Answer: C

Answer: The patient probably does not have any thyroid problems.
This patient is critically sick. In severe illness, the pituitary secretes less TSH, which results in a low or low-normal FT_4. However, T_4 is not the active hormone; T_3 is active. In severe illness, T_3 levels are greatly suppressed. With the T_4 being lower, there is less T_4 available to be converted into T_3. However, there is still considerable T_4 present. In order to protect the body from the active T_3 hormone, the T_4 is converted into an inactive hormone called reverse T_3 (rT_3). Levels of rT_3 are rarely measured, but if it was measured in this patient, it would be greatly elevated.

This patient is most likely euthyroid, but also very sick. He does not have hypothyroidism or hyperthyroidism, either primary or secondary. There is no need to act on his abnormal thyroid tests; instead treat his underlying illness.

Board Testing Point: Recognize that thyroid function tests are not likely to be accurate in patients with severe acute illnesses (especially if they are hospitalized in ICUs).

310. Answer: B

Answer: Refer him for a thyroid fine-needle biopsy and aspiration (FNA).
This patient is euthyroid, but with a thyroid nodule. Perform a thyroid FNA yourself, or refer him to someone who can. If the biopsy is not conclusive, then most would repeat it. If the lesion is hot and the patient is euthyroid, they can either be followed or, if the patient is hyperthyroid, radioiodine therapy or surgery can be recommended. A near-total thyroidectomy would be needed only if cancer was present. Many physicians in the past have tried to shrink nodules with thyroxine, thinking that exogenous thyroxine will lower the TSH, which will reduce the growth stimulation to the nodule. Unfortunately, studies have shown this not to be the case; thyroxine should not be given in the hope of shrinking a nodule. Considering how easy and safe a thyroid biopsy is, it would be inappropriate to just follow him. Though the vast majority of nodules are benign, cancer cannot be excluded by simply watching the nodule.

Board Testing Point: Be familiar with how to work up an isolated thyroid nodule in a euthyroid patient.

311. Answer: A

Answer: Begin antithyroid medication now and postpone the surgery until he is euthyroid or nearly so. This question requires you to understand the dangers of hyperthyroidism in a patient going into surgery. This patient has signs of hyperthyroidism, which is verified by laboratory tests. In a patient with hyperthyroidism, any kind of surgery can trigger a severe uncompensated hyperthyroidism (thyroid storm), which can be fatal. Treatment of the hyperthyroidism should be initiated before the surgery takes place. The question of whether to postpone the operation is a little more problematic and depends on whether the surgery is emergent, urgent, or routine. Obviously, if the surgery is an emergency and cannot be postponed, ask the anesthesiologist to administer iodine to inhibit thyroid hormone synthesis (this can be administered as intravenous radiocontrast agents), β-blockers to block the adrenergic effects of hyperthyroidism, and glucocorticoids to protect from the stress of hyperthyroidism and to inhibit the conversion of T_4 to T_3. If the surgery is routine and can be delayed, as in this case, the patient should be started on antithyroid medications, and the operation should be postponed until the patient is rendered euthyroid or nearly euthyroid. An operation that is urgent, but not emergent, can be postponed for a limited amount of time. During this interval, begin antithyroid medications (PTU or methimazole), iodide, and β-blockers. Though the patient will probably not be euthyroid before surgery, his hyperthyroidism will at least be lessened in severity and may protect him from developing thyroid storm.

Board Testing Point: Recognize the dangers of operating on a patient who is clinically hyperthyroid.

312. Answer: D

Answer: Order TSH and FT_4, suspecting hypothyroidism due to postpartum thyroiditis.
Many young mothers will report postpartum depression, which will resolve on its own. However, some of these cases of postpartum depression may actually signify postpartum thyroiditis. The typical presentation is an uneventful pregnancy and delivery followed by an initial period of hyperthyroidism lasting for about 1 month, which is followed by a protracted period of hypothyroidism lasting for many months and sometimes for a year. The initial period of hyperthyroidism is easily tolerated. After all, the woman will have considerable energy and will lose weight more easily. However, she will soon develop hypothyroidism. Once you verify with TSH and FT_4 that she is hypothyroid, begin treating her with thyroxine. Her hypothyroidism is not likely to be permanent, so follow her monthly and adjust the thyroxine dose as needed, ultimately discontinuing it.

Board Testing Point: Recognize the clinical characteristics of postpartum thyroiditis.

313. Answer: B

Answer: He has diabetes and must talk with a diabetes educator and dietitian to begin a diet, exercise program, and metformin.
He fulfills 2 diagnostic criteria for diabetes. The full set of criteria includes: 1) random glucose ≥ 200 mg/dL with symptoms (polyuria, polydipsia, or unexplained weight loss); 2) fasting glucose ≥ 126 mg/dL; and 3) 2-hour 75 g oral glucose tolerance test (OGTT) ≥ 200 mg/dL. Now that you have diagnosed him, you must next determine whether he has Type 1 or Type 2 diabetes. He most likely has Type 2, because he is overweight, and there is no mention of metabolic decompensation. You must now determine whether to treat and, if so, how. There is no question about it—you must intervene immediately. There is nothing to benefit from waiting. However, in the absence of metabolic decompensation and severe hyperglycemia, it is most prudent to begin with lifestyle changes. He must be educated on the importance of an exercise program, and he must learn how to eat a healthful diet. Current recommendations now include beginning metformin in all patients with their initial diagnosis of Type 2 diabetes. This is because of the difficulty in achieving and sustaining glycemic control and achieving significant weight loss.

Board Testing Point: Know the laboratory criteria for diagnosing diabetes mellitus, and recognize that metformin is now an initial therapy in addition to diet and exercise.

314. Answer: B

Answer: Reduce her evening NPH insulin and follow closely.
Her symptoms of vivid nightmares and waking in a cold sweat are compatible with nocturnal hypoglycemia. The most likely explanation for the early morning hyperglycemia is that the nocturnal hypoglycemia is causing the contra-insular hormones (glucagon, cortisol, growth hormone, and epinephrine) to be secreted. Many Type 1 diabetics lose the ability to secrete glucagon in response to hypoglycemia, but the remaining hormones are unaffected. These hormones will raise the glucose level. However, insulin-deficient persons such as this patient do not have the ability to make their own insulin to control the hyperglycemic effect of the contra-insular hormones, and her morning fasting glucose levels are elevated. Every patient taking insulin needs to perform self-monitoring of their blood glucose levels. They should check their glucose before and 2 hours after every meal, at bedtime, and in the middle of the night around 3 a.m. Of course it's impractical to constantly check glucose levels this often on a daily basis. One alternative is to have patients check their glucose level twice every day, choosing different times each day so that the log book will have some numbers at each time point. The 3 a.m. glucose level should be checked at least once each month, but doesn't need to be checked much more frequently—unless the patient is having evidence of nocturnal hypoglycemia or has changed the insulin regimen. Once this patient no longer has hypoglycemia, the insulin can always be carefully and slowly increased.

It is inappropriate to begin an anxiolytic rather than decreasing the insulin. Hypoglycemia can be life-threatening. Increasing her evening insulin further could be fatal. There is no evidence that she has insulin resistance in addition to her insulin deficiency, and adding an insulin sensitizer is inappropriate. Switching her to a 70/30 premix is also inappropriate. The goal of treating a Type 1 diabetic is to replace the insulin in a physiologic way. Her insulin regimen is already physiologic by offering basal coverage with NPH twice daily and bolus coverage with a rapid-acting insulin analog with each meal.

Board Testing Point: Recognize the clinical manifestations of nocturnal hypoglycemia due to excess administration of insulin before bedtime, in an attempt to lower morning glucose values.

315. Answer: C

Answer: Add an ACE inhibitor or an angiotensin-receptor blocker (ARB).
The random urine screen indicates microalbuminuria. Normal albumin excretion is < 30 mg/day, microalbuminuria is 30–300 mg/day, and macroalbuminuria is > 300 mg/day. Collecting an accurate 24-hour urine is difficult and problematic. Fortunately, creatinine excretion is somewhat consistent when adjusted for standard body surface area. This has led to use of the albumin:creatinine ratio in a random spot urine as a surrogate marker. A normal ratio is < 30 µg/mg, microalbuminuria is 30–300 µg/mg, and macroalbuminuria is > 300 µg/mg. If the ratio is only slightly above normal, it is best to repeat the random urine or to ask for a 24-hour urine to better quantitate the albumin excretion. In addition, any urinary tract infection must be completely resolved before checking for albuminuria. His ratio is well within the range of microalbuminuria, and there is no suspicion of a urinary tract infection. Once a diabetic has microalbuminuria, the patient must be treated. The goal of treatment is to slow the progression of the nephropathy in an attempt to prevent end-stage renal disease. Several studies have shown that an ACE inhibitor is an excellent drug for this purpose, and some recent studies have shown that ARBs may be just as beneficial. The best course of action for this patient is to begin one of these drugs.

The patient is certainly doing a good job by watching his diet, consistently walking, and losing weight. He should be praised for this, but he also needs treatment for the nephropathy. There is no reason to increase his statin, since the LDL is less than 100 mg/dL (goal). A calcium channel blocker may be useful for hypertension, but is not the initial drug of choice in diabetics with nephropathy. Likewise, a diuretic can be useful for blood pressure control, but is not the initial drug of choice in a diabetic with nephropathy.

Board Testing Point: Recognize that following microalbuminuria is important in diabetics, and once it occurs it is necessary to start an ACE inhibitor or ARB.

316. Answer: D

Answer: Primary hyperparathyroidism.
The PTH is elevated along with the calcium. Normally, an elevated calcium would suppress the PTH level. His PTH is elevated in the face of hypercalcemia and thus represents primary hyperparathyroidism. The only other rare differential diagnosis is FHH (familial hypocalciuric hyercalcemia), which could be excluded by checking a 24-hour urine for calcium and asking about familial history of hypercalcemia.

His vitamin D levels are elevated, but this is due to both his primary hyperparathyroidism and his use of vitamin supplements. Vitamin A intoxication can cause hypercalcemia, but no vitamin A levels are given in this question, and his primary hyperparathyroidism is a better explanation. Pseudopseudohypoparathyroidism refers to a specific phenotype (shortened 4th and 5th metacarpals) with normal calcium and parathyroid hormone levels. His labs rule out such a diagnosis. Secondary hyperparathyroidism refers to the normally elevated levels of parathyroid hormone in the face of hypocalcemia. Low calcium levels will stimulate the parathyroid glands to secrete extra hormone, which will stimulate the conversion of 25-OH-vitamin D into 1,25-$(OH)_2$-vitamin D. His calcium is elevated, so he cannot have secondary hyperparathyroidism.

Board Testing Point: Recognize the laboratory features of primary hyperparathyroidism.

317. Answer: B

Answer: Vitamin D deficiency.
This lady has probably had hypocalcemia for quite some time and came to medical attention only because she experienced an osteoporotic hip fracture. An extremely common cause of hypocalcemia is vitamin D deficiency, and she exhibits a classic presentation. Her 25-OH-vitamin D level is low, reflecting both her poor diet and her low exposure to sunlight due to her reluctance to leave the house. Hypocalcemia normally gives rise to an elevated parathyroid hormone level (secondary hyperparathyroidism) and this in turn stimulates the conversion of 25-OH-vitamin D to 1,25-$(OH)_2$-vitamin D. Unfortunately, her levels of 25-OH-vitamin D are already low, and her conversion to 1,25-$(OH)_2$-vitamin D is thus impaired. The phosphate level is low because of the hyperparathyroidism, which stimulates renal excretion of phosphates.

While hypomagnesemia can cause hypocalcemia due to impaired secretion of parathyroid hormone, her hypermagnesemia is not contributing. Hyperphosphatemia may cause hypocalcemia because of local precipitation of calcium-phosphate salts. Her hypophosphatemia is not the cause of the hypocalcemia. Thiazide diuretics are associated with hypercalcemia, not hypocalcemia. Primary hyperparathyroidism causes hypercalcemia, not hypocalcemia.

Board Testing Point: Recognize the clinical features of vitamin D deficiency in an elderly homebound patient.

318. Answer: C

Answer: Discontinue his oral agents for glycemic control and switch him to insulin.
This question requires you to know that triglyceride levels are very dependent upon glycemic control. This patient has gained a significant amount of weight, and his insulin resistance has worsened to the point that he is not controlled on the combination of a thiazolidinedione, metformin, and a rapid-acting secretagogue, despite taking the maximum allowable doses. At this point, he must be switched to insulin. His triglyceride level was much better 6 months ago when his glycemic control was better. It is safe to assume that the increase in triglyceride levels is due to his worsening control. This scenario is commonly seen with diabetic patients. Before specifically targeting his triglyceride levels, his glycemic control must first be improved.

Adding a fibrate to a statin is controversial. Though some physicians do it, the combination is not approved by the FDA at the time of this writing. A fibrate could certainly be used once the statin was discontinued, but a fibrate is not as good an agent at lowering LDL cholesterol. His LDL was 170 mg/dL in the past. It is unlikely that his LDL will remain controlled once he has been switched from a statin to a fibrate. An α-glucosidase inhibitor is expected to lower HbA1c by about 0.5 percentage points. This will not provide enough control for his hyperglycemia. Adding a second statin will not help the situation. If anything, this will increase his risk of an adverse event.

Board Testing Point: Recognize that poor glucose control results in worsening of hypertriglyceridemia.

319. Answer: A

Answer: Begin dexamethasone 4 mg IV and order an ACTH stimulation test.
There is a strong suspicion that this patient has adrenal insufficiency and is having an adrenal crisis. She is hypovolemic with a hyperkalemic metabolic acidosis. The hypotension responded well to saline fluids. The thin body habitus and loss of axillary and pubic hair imply a chronic adrenal insufficiency. The flight delay may have caused stress for some reason that she was not able to cope with because of the adrenal insufficiency. This may have been what tipped her over the edge. Whether she really has an adrenal crisis or not is not the issue. It is more important to begin treatment than it is to prove your suspicion. The treatment is to give her

intravenous glucocorticoids as soon as possible. But which glucocorticoid should you give? Remember, you do not yet have proof of the adrenal insufficiency. You can start treatment based on a suspicion, but you must also pursue a diagnosis. The diagnostic workup begins with an ACTH stimulation test. To do this, order a baseline serum cortisol level, administer 1 ampule of ACTH, and repeat the cortisol level 30 minutes later. The important thing to remember is that the assay for cortisol will cross-react with most other glucocorticoids and also pick up prednisone, methylprednisolone, and especially hydrocortisone since it is cortisol under a different name. If any of these are administered, how will you know what her endogenous production of cortisol really is? The solution is to administer a glucocorticoid that does not interfere with the cortisol assay, such as dexamethasone. She needs a glucocorticoid to save her life; begin dexamethasone immediately. If her adrenal function proves to be okay, you can easily stop the steroid. To check her adrenal function, check for her response to ACTH. If the cortisol level is greater than 20 µg/dL, her adrenal reserve is intact and you can stop the dexamethasone. If the ACTH stimulation test shows adrenal insufficiency, stop the dexamethasone and switch her to hydrocortisone. This is the actual cortisol molecule, and it has an advantage over the other glucocorticoids. Hydrocortisone (cortisol) is primarily a glucocorticoid, but it also has some mineralocorticoid activity that will help with her electrolytes.

The other answers are incorrect because a glucocorticoid other than dexamethasone should not be used for the above reasons. Hypothyroidism is unlikely, so starting thyroxine is not indicated. Once her adrenal crisis has resolved, you can reevaluate her.

Board Testing Point: Recognize the clinical manifestations of adrenal insufficiency and how to manage it appropriately in an emergency setting.

---

320. Answer: D

Answer: Vitamin A intoxication.
His 25-OH-vitamin D levels may be mildly elevated from excess supplementation, but the body regulates the active 1,25-$(OH)_2$-vitamin D, which is low due to low iPTH. The real culprit may be vitamin A intoxication, which increases intestinal absorption of calcium and stimulates osteoclasts to release calcium and phosphorus from bone. The elevated calcium suppresses PTH, and the reduced PTH results in less urinary clearance of phosphorus.

Board Testing Point: Recognize the clinical features and laboratory findings of vitamin A intoxication.

---

321. Answer: E

Answer: Thyroid scan and uptake.
You need to know thyroid **function**, not just its anatomy. The absence of symptoms due to mass effect from the thyroid—e.g., no recurrent laryngeal nerve impingement (i.e., no voice change, weakness, or "gravelly" sound), and no dysphagia or dyspnea—excludes the need for anatomic studies: MRI, CT, ultrasound, and scan. By obtaining a thyroid scan and uptake (which reveal the gland's **functional** ability to concentrate I-131), you will find diminished uptake except in the left lower pole of the thyroid where there is a "hot" nodule.

Board Testing Point: Recognize the clinical features of hyperthyroidism and determine the next best test to help diagnose the etiology.

---

322. Answer: A

Answer: Atorvastatin.
The point here is that he needs LDL treated and, if possible, HDL raised. He is already exercising, which is an excellent means to raise HDL.

Board Testing Point: Recognize that a statin is the best choice for treatment of an elevated LDL cholesterol.

323. Answer: C

Answer: Basal plasma ACTH and cortisol ACTH stimulation test.
This is a classic presentation for Addison disease. She has fatigue, asthenia and listlessness, and recurrent flu-like illnesses. Further history may be that of a family history of autoimmune endocrine disorders (Type 1 diabetes, Hashimoto disease, Graves disease) or of tuberculosis she acquired overseas (if it had been left untreated). A basal plasma ACTH and cortisol ACTH stimulation test should be done next. If the cortisol is low and the ACTH is high, it indicates primary adrenal insufficiency (Addison disease). Screening for other autoimmune endocrine disorders is reasonable, but not a priority. This is not the history of bulimia, so a dental screening for enamel etching due to vomiting is not necessary. Treatment should be a corticosteroid and mineralocorticoid, since the aldosterone-producing cells are often involved to some extent.

Board Testing Point: Recognize the clinical features of adrenal insufficiency and know how to begin the diagnostic workup.

324. Answer: D

Answer: Adrenal cancer.
This question asks you to know that 2 things—late onset and rapid progression of androgenization—mean cancer. The ovary is the major source of measured testosterone in the woman; the adrenal is the major producer of DHEA, so extraordinarily high DHEA-S means adrenal cancer. To evaluate hirsutism requires DHEA-S and testosterone. If the hirsutism is milder and insidious with symptoms beginning in puberty or the early 20s, it is more likely due to PCOS; in which case, LH: FSH ratio over 2.5 along with high normal or above normal testosterone occurs. Two unfortunate things about treatment for adrenal carcinoma: it demands prompt excision, and it has a poor prognosis.

Board Testing Point: Recognize the clinical and laboratory features of adrenal carcinoma.

325. Answer: B

Answer: Klinefelter syndrome.
This exam points toward eunuchoid development with span greater than height, which is compatible with late epiphyseal closure due to underproduction of testosterone; and the gynecomastia also points toward relatively insufficient testosterone production. The key is the small (usually described as firm) testes and gynecomastia, which point to Klinefelter syndrome. Kallmann syndrome is not correct, because congenital hypogonadotropic hypogonadism has low amounts of both estrogens and testosterone, so gynecomastia does not develop. Pituitary adenoma and prolactinoma do not have the skeletal manifestations listed. Hereditary small gonad syndrome is not a true syndrome.

Board Testing Point: Recognize the clinical features of Klinefelter syndrome.

326. Answer: E

Answer: Increase the supper insulin lispro, and decrease the bedtime NPH.
You are asked to recognize that erratic fasting glucoses may represent unrecognized nocturnal hypoglycemia, and so you should cut her bedtime NPH.

Board Testing Point: Recognize the clinical features of nocturnal hypoglycemia, and that reducing evening longer-acting insulin will prevent rebound morning glucoses as well as hypoglycemic symptoms during the night.

327. Answer: A

Answer: Stop the prednisone abruptly.
A week or less of high-dose glucocorticoids would not be expected to suppress the hypothalamic-pituitary-adrenal axis to the point that steroids need to be continued while waiting for return of function. Two weeks of high-dose steroids would certainly suppress the axis and require continuation of a replacement dose while checking for return of function. The period between 1 week and 2 weeks is very variable, and replacement dose should be continued to err on the side of caution.

Board Testing Point: Recognize that short-term high-dose corticosteroid therapy does not suppress the hypothalamic-pituitary-adrenal axis.

328. Answer: A

Answer: Metformin.
For a consistently elevated fasting glucose with diet modification, metformin is indicated to diminish hepatic gluconeogenesis. It is the first-step treatment for Type 2 diabetes. She now has had 2 fasting blood glucoses ≥ 126 mg/dL, and you have made the diagnosis of Type 2 diabetes. She should be started on metformin now if there are no contraindications (most important to know is that for women, creatinine must be < 1.4 mg/dL and for men < 1.5 mg/dL).

Board Testing Point: Recognize that the initial treatment for Type 2 diabetes mellitus has always included diet and weight loss, but now metformin is recommended as initial therapy as well.

329. Answer: C

Answer: Symptoms of hypoglycemia, low serum glucose, and symptom relief with glucose.
This patient scenario leads you to understand causes of hypoglycemia and to differentiate between fasting (insulinoma) and post-prandial (dumping syndrome and "reactive") hypoglycemia. Once you discriminate between hypoglycemia that occurs in the fasting state (due to insulin excess, either endogenous or exogenous) and hypoglycemia that occurs after eating, the correct diagnosis is post-gastrectomy syndrome. Also, it is necessary to remember that Whipple's triad of hypoglycemic symptoms occurs during periods of low serum glucose and is relieved by a source of sugar.

Board Testing Point: Know the meaning of Whipple's triad.

330. Answer: E

Answer: Paget disease.
Paget disease causes an asymptomatic elevation of alkaline phosphatase. Since the patients can be asymptomatic or have aching that is similar in quality to the pain of degenerative joint disease (DJD), indications for intervention are important to know: encroachment on neuro-foramen, CHF from increased blood flow, threat to weight-bearing bones, and pain are reasons for treatment.

Board Testing Point: Recognize the clinical and laboratory features of Paget disease.

331. Answer: D

Answer: Graves disease.
In this case, realize that Graves disease is unlikely! The thyrotoxic phase of subacute and silent thyroiditis is associated with an inflammatory breakdown and release of stored thyroid hormone, which will feed back onto the hypothalamus and anterior pituitary to inhibit TSH secretion. This will produce a low RAIU for a while. Struma ovarii, remember, consists of ectopic hyperfunctioning autonomous thyroid tissue—like in a teratoma, which also will result in a low RAIU in the thyroid (however, if the pelvis is scanned, it would show an **increased** uptake here). Iodine-induced thyrotoxicosis will generally occur in the face of a preexisting dysfunctional thyroid. We see this mainly in someone who is coming from a country with **low** iodine intake, to the USA with our **high** iodine intakes.

Board Testing Point: Recognize the clinical and laboratory features associated with hyperthyroidism and the use of a radioactive iodine uptake test to help differentiate the etiology.

332. Answer: C

Answer: Do nothing at this point.
This guy has familial hypocalciuric hypercalcemia (FHH), also known as benign familial hypercalcemia. This consists of an elevated serum calcium, normal or low serum phosphorus, a normal or high serum PTH, a slightly elevated magnesium, and a low urinary calcium excretion. This is inherited as an autosomal dominant disorder of chromosomes 3 or 19. No therapy is required.

Surgery will not correct the hypercalcemia. The other thing to be careful about is that these patients can be misdiagnosed as having hyperparathyroidism if the urinary calcium is not measured. Untreated, these patients generally remain asymptomatic without evidence of renal calculi, HTN, or other problems with hypercalcemia.

Board Testing Point: Recognize the clinical features of familial hypocalciuric hypercalcemia.

333. Answer: B

Answer: The patient likely has tertiary hyperparathyroidism.
This is seen commonly in renal patients where the parathyroid glands become autonomous. The hypercalcemia develops gradually over time and is rarely life-threatening. It is associated with osteitis fibrosa. It can be treated with aluminum "binders." Finally, parathyroid hormone half-life is actually **increased** in renal insufficiency.

Board Testing Point: Recognize the findings of tertiary hyperparathyroidism.

334. Answer: A

Answer: Radioactive iodine uptake.
This postpartum female has symptoms and lab work suggesting hyperthyroidism. The most common cause in this setting would be postpartum thyroiditis. The most definitive test to rule out the alternative diagnosis of Graves disease would be a 24-hour radioactive iodine uptake. Patients with Graves disease have a high 24-hour radioiodine uptake, whereas patients with acute or subacute thyroiditis have a very low radioiodine uptake. The radioiodine uptake test cannot be performed if she is nursing. In this instance, most would consider watchful waiting. If she has postpartum thyroiditis, her symptoms will improve; if she has Graves', she will worsen or not improve.

Board Testing Point: Know how to differentiate postpartum thyroiditis from Graves disease in a woman who is postpartum and not breastfeeding.

335. Answer: D

Answer: Interaction between levothyroxine sodium and $FeSO_4$.
This patient has a history of hypothyroidism treated with levothyroxine. She develops iron-deficiency anemia and is started on iron. She then develops symptoms and signs of hypothyroidism: dry skin, elevated cholesterol, constipation, and muscle pain. The reason for her hypothyroidism is poor absorption of the levothyroxine she is taking due to an interaction between the oral iron and the levothyroxine.

Board Testing Point: Recognize the drug interaction between iron and levothyroxine.

336. Answer: B

Answer: 50-year-old man with fasting plasma glucose of 113 mg/dL.
A fasting glucose between 100–125 is impaired fasting glucose and considered prediabetes.

An HbA1c of more than 6.5% is diagnostic of diabetes. Using 75 grams of glucose in an oral glucose tolerance test, a blood glucose between 140 and 199 is consistent with prediabetes. A glucose > 200 after a 75 g OGTT is diagnostic of diabetes. A 2-hour post challenge glucose < 140 is normal. A fasting glucose between 70 and 99 is normal.

Board Testing Point: Know how to distinguish prediabetes and diabetes.

337. Answer: B

Answer: Her insulin requirements will decrease by 50%.
During pregnancy, a patient with diabetes requires ~ 50% more insulin due to increased resistance from placental hormones. This increased requirement is gone immediately after delivery and her insulin requirements will decrease by at least 50% in the first 24 hours after delivery. Her blood glucoses will need to be monitored carefully during that time period. Again, insulin requirements increase during pregnancy and decline after delivery. She is insulin-dependent, and stopping insulin could lead to ketoacidosis. Babies of diabetic mothers are at risk for hypoglycemia in the immediate period after birth.

Board Testing Point: Anticipate the changes in insulin requirements during the first 24 hours after delivery in a patient with Type 1 diabetes.

338. Answer: D

Answer: Repeat ultrasound in 1 year.
Nodules smaller than 10 mm do not require fine needle aspiration, and the ultrasound should be repeated in 1 year to determine if there has been a change in nodule size. A technetium scan is not necessary, because the TSH is normal and thus no reason to differentiate between a hypofunctioning and hyperfunctioning nodule. TPO antibodies may be elevated because autoimmune thyroid disease is common, but the antibody titer is not useful in evaluation of a nodule.

Board Testing Point: Know how to evaluate an incidentally discovered thyroid nodule.

339. Answer: B

Answer: Lower the dose of methimazole.
For women who are hyperthyroid during pregnancy, it is important to keep the free T_4 at the upper end of the normal range and TSH at the lower range. A low or low normal free T_4 could lead to fetal hypothyroidism and fetal thyroid enlargement, which might compromise delivery. PTU is not recommended after the 1st trimester, and radioactive iodine should always be avoided during pregnancy. The correct answer is to lower the dose of methimazole to achieve a free T_4 in the upper range of normal and TSH at the lower range. Surgery is not indicated for uncomplicated Graves' during pregnancy.

Board Testing Point: Know the management of hyperthyroidism during pregnancy.

340. Answer: C

Answer: Thyroglobulin.
The suppressed TSH indicates that she either has endogenous or exogenous hyperthyroidism and a free T_4, T_3; and total T_4 will be elevated in both unless the patient has T_3 toxicosis (endogenous or exogenous). The low uptake on the scan is consistent with either thyroiditis or exogenous T_4. Thyroglobulin will be elevated with thyroiditis, because the gland is inflamed, but will not be elevated with exogenous use of T_4 because the gland is suppressed. An ultrasound is not designed to assess thyroid function.

Board Testing Point: Know how to distinguish between exogenous and endogenous hyperthyroidism.

341. Answer: C

Answer: Weight loss.
The prevention of diabetes in at-risk patients is a key goal of primary care providers. Numerous large studies on the prevention of diabetes in patients have been conducted. Smoking cessation has been examined and may be helpful, but no definitive data have been shown. Thiazolidinediones have been shown to at least delay the onset of diabetes and possibly prevent its onset; cost and side effect concerns have limited their use in this capacity. The most significant and well-studied interventions involve diet, exercise changes, and metformin. The Diabetes Prevention Program (DPP) was a large RCT that compared lifestyle changes with metformin and placebo in examining incidence of diabetes. Lifestyle changes were significantly better than metformin, while both were significantly better than placebo. In certain populations, metformin may be recommended for treatment to prevent diabetes, but it is not the most effective therapy.

Board Testing Point: Recognize that weight loss is the most effective intervention to prevent diabetes.

HEMATOLOGY

342. Answer: B

Answer: Protein C deficiency.
Coumadin-induced skin necrosis has been well described in patients with protein C deficiency. The skin lesions most commonly occur on the breasts, buttocks, and legs. The penis is also a described site. The theory is that an imbalance in homeostasis occurs, favoring thrombosis during the early phases of coumadin administration. We know that protein C has a short half-life of about 14 hours compared to some of the vitamin K-dependent factors such as Factor X—and a rapid drop in the protein C concentration could produce this scenario.

Board Testing Point: Recognize the association of protein C deficiency with coumadin-induced skin necrosis.

343. Answer: C

Answer: Alpha-thalassemia trait.
This occurs when people have deletion of 2 of the 4 alpha-chain genes. These individuals tend to have a microcytic and slightly hypochromic red cell, but without significant anemia or hemolysis. Hemoglobin electrophoresis can be normal or may show a decreased amount of hemoglobin A_2. All of the other abnormalities listed would have microcytosis, but the hemoglobin electrophoresis would be abnormal.

Board Testing Point: Recognize the laboratory features in alpha-thalassemia trait.

344. Answer: B

Answer: Intravascular hemolysis has likely occurred.
This presentation is consistent with a delayed transfusion reaction. Immediate transfusion reactions that would manifest as intravascular hemolysis are most commonly due to ABO incompatibility. Usually these are due to clerical error. Fever, malaise, and a drop in hematocrit 1 week after red cell transfusion are typical of delayed transfusion reactions, which are usually mediated by antibodies to Rh unless the patient is Rh-negative, in which case it is mediated by antibodies to anti-Duffy, anti-Kell, or anti-Kidd. These antibodies coat the donor red cells, which results in a positive direct Coombs test. Less commonly, the donor's plasma could contain antibodies that might react with the recipient's cells.

Board Testing Point: Recognize the clinical features of a delayed transfusion reaction.

345. Answer: C

Answer: Aspirin.
She has von Willebrand disease (vWD), and using aspirin would further aggravate her ability to aggregate platelet response. The other drugs listed are not contraindicated in vWD.

Board Testing Point: Recognize the clinical and laboratory features of von Willebrand disease, and know that aspirin should be avoided in these patients.

346. Answer: C

Answer: Myelodysplastic syndrome.
Myelodysplastic syndrome is usually seen in elderly patients (she is quite young) and is characterized by **high** MCVs and hypercellular bone marrows. Iron deficiency anemia will give you a low MCV with anemia, as she has. In anemia of chronic disease you usually have a normal MCV, but it can be low on occasion. The thalassemias (alpha and beta) will produce a microcytic anemia, as she has. Sideroblastic anemia is rare but would have these findings.

Board Testing Point: Recognize the clinical features of myelodysplastic syndrome.

347. Answer: A

Answer: Hepatic venography or magnetic resonance (MR) venography.
He most likely has polycythemia rubra vera with the presence of primary erythrocytosis with organomegaly. A complication of this disorder is hypercoagulability, with hepatic vein thrombosis being a particular problem seen. Hepatic vein thrombosis would lead to Budd-Chiari syndrome, where you would have a grossly enlarged liver with severe ascites. The best way to diagnosis this is by hepatic venography, MR venography, or liver biopsy, where you would look for sinusoidal dilatation. Ultrasound with Dopplers or a CT scan of the hepatic circulation would also be helpful as a screening diagnostic tool. The hepatic venogram is the gold standard, but in many institutions MRI venography is replacing it because of its noninvasive character.

Board Testing Point: Recognize the clinical features of polycythemia rubra vera and the association with thrombosis of the hepatic vein.

348. Answer: B

Answer: Normal levels of protein C rules out the disease.
This is **incorrect** about protein C deficiency! Protein C is an anticoagulant that inactivates clotting Factors V and VII. When deficient, it can lead to thrombosis commonly of the lower extremity deep veins as well as the iliofemoral or mesenteric veins. The majority are spontaneous while the rest occur in association with a stress such as surgery or pregnancy. It is inherited as an autosomal dominant disease. Two forms of the disease exist: 1) normal levels of protein C (but a biologically dysfunctional protein); 2) deficient levels of protein C. Therefore, just measuring the level of protein C will not "rule out" the disease. You must also measure "tests of function." Besides the inherited form, acquired protein C deficiency can occur. This can happen with DIC, severe liver disease, nephrotic syndrome, etc.

Board Testing Point: Recognize features associated with protein C deficiency.

349. Answer: E

Answer: Salvage chemo/immunotherapy, followed by autologous stem cell transplantation.
Hodgkin disease that relapses, especially if it is not primary refractory, can potentially be cured by autologous bone marrow transplantation after salvage chemotherapy.

Rituximab, a chimeric monoclonal antibody against CD20, is usually not used in classical Hodgkin disease because it tends to be CD20-negative. Brentuximab is a monoclonal antibody conjugate against CD30, and though it is a good salvage option, needs to be consolidated with autologous transplant. Repeat ABVD alone most likely will not cure the patient, and there is also the lifetime maximum dose of doxorubicin to consider. Whatever the salvage regimen is used, this young man will need to be worked up and referred for an autologous transplant, preferably in a complete remission.

Board Testing Point: Know the role of transplantation in relapsed Hodgkin disease as a potential curative option and appropriate referral.

350. Answer: D

Answer: Multiple myeloma.
She has multiple myeloma, which is the primary culprit of her bone pain, weight loss, night sweats, and splenomegaly. In addition, the elevated ESR, anemia, renal failure, positive SPEP, Bence-Jones proteinuria, and lytic lesions on skeletal x-rays all support this diagnosis.

Although most elderly females have OA of their hands, the constitutional symptoms and abnormal labs are not seen with OA. Amyloid would have an elevated ESR, anemia, and renal failure, but not an abnormal SPEP, Bence-Jones proteins, nor lytic lesions. Gout in postmenopausal females would most likely be polyarticular with hands, knees, ankles, and/or podagra as the presentation, not weight loss, night sweats, nor splenomegaly.

Board Testing Point: Recognize the clinical features of multiple myeloma.

351. Answer: E

Answer: Hydration and analgesia.
She is having a sickle cell pain crisis that frequently can be precipitated by an upper respiratory infection or dehydration. It can be very difficult to distinguish from a crisis and an acute abdomen, so vigilance must be observed. Hydration is initially the key! Hydroxyurea may reduce the incidence of sickle crises by increasing synthesis of fetal hemoglobin, but has no role in an acute crisis. Antibiotics would be administered only if an infection was documented. Chest syndrome is something to be very concerned about in this patient and would require aggressive monitoring of her condition.

Board Testing Point: Recognize the initial management of a sickle cell pain crisis.

352. Answer: A

Answer: Stop PTU and schedule a follow-up appointment.
She most likely has severe neutropenia as an idiosyncratic reaction to PTU. She is at risk for an overwhelming, life-threatening infection; however, at the moment, without signs of fever or other signs of infection, she can be followed as an outpatient. Steroids are not useful in this setting. You would never continue the offending drug. Almost always, severe drug-induced neutropenia reverses fairly quickly, and therefore consideration for bone marrow transplant is not indicated at this point.

Board Testing Point: Recognize the clinical characteristics of drug-induced neutropenia and know how to manage this complication appropriately.

353. Answer: D

Answer: Plasmapheresis.
This woman has thrombocytopenic purpura (TTP). You can put this together very easily: Hemolytic anemia with fragmented red cells, thrombocytopenia, fever, mental status changes, and renal dysfunction **without** evidence of disseminated intravascular coagulation (DIC) is classic for TTP. Plasmapheresis or exchange transfusion is the preferred treatment.

Board Testing Point: Identify the clinical features of thrombocytopenic purpura.

354. Answer: C

Answer: She has developed alloantibodies in her serum.
Patients who receive a large number of transfusions frequently will develop a large panel of alloantibodies. This makes it difficult to type and match appropriate blood for these patients. The presence of these antibodies may or may not produce hemolysis if blood containing a potential target antigen is transfused; however, blood banks will not allow transfusion of these products unless it is an emergency situation.

Board Testing Point: Recognize the findings associated with the development of alloantibodies after multiple transfusions in a patient with sickle cell disease.

355. Answer: A

Answer: Severe hypokalemia.
Severe hypokalemia may occur early in the course of therapy. This represents a marked increase in potassium utilization during the production of new hematopoietic cells. Reticulocytosis is usually brisk and is a hallmark of correct diagnosis and treatment of this disease.

Board Testing Point: Recognize that treatment of an anemia may result in the development of hypokalemia.

356. Answer: D

Answer: Folate in large doses can correct the megaloblastic anemia, but it does not correct the neurologic abnormalities.
Pernicious anemia is a condition that leads to decreased red blood cell production due to vitamin B_{12} deficiency, leading to megaloblastic anemia. The mechanism by which this occurs is thought to be an autoimmune process leading to production of antibodies to the parietal cells in the stomach, which make intrinsic factor. Antiparietal cell antibodies are common and seen in 90% of those with pernicious anemia. Gastrin levels are usually elevated in those with pernicious anemia. Oral folic acid can usually correct or prevent the megaloblatic anemia of perniocus anemia. However, since B_{12} is also involved in neurological function and its deficiency can cause neurological symptoms like sensory and motor neuropathy, which cannot be reversed by folic acid supplementation. Thus, it could mask the underlying disease and allow the development or progression of neurological deterioration, if diagnosis depended on the presence of anemic symptoms alone.

Board Testing Point: Recognize the clinical features of pernicious anemia.

357. Answer: E

Answer: Abnormalities of iron metabolism with trapping of iron in macrophages.
Actually, there are several factors thought to be responsible for the hypoproliferative state of red cell production:

1) Abnormalities of iron metabolism with trapping of iron in macrophages. This results in reduced plasma iron levels (hypoferremia), making iron relatively unavailable for new hemoglobin synthesis.
2) Inability of the morphologically normal marrow to increase erythropoiesis in response to anemia. Serum erythropoietin (EPO) levels are somewhat elevated, but there is virtually no increase in erythropoiesis, perhaps due to increased apoptotic death of red cell precursors.
3) A relative decrease in EPO production. The inverse relationship between hematocrit levels and serum EPO seen in most anemic conditions is not maintained in anemia of chronic disease.

In addition, patients with anemia of chronic disease have lower levels of EPO than do patients with iron deficiency and a similar degree of anemia. Shortening of red cell life span may occur in cases of acute inflammation characterized by increased erythrophagocytosis. The anemia of chronic disease is usually a normochromic, normocytic anemia. Bone marrow examination will show normal red cell maturation. Hemolysis does not typically occur. Hemoglobin synthesis is usually normal also. Patients most often have a low serum iron and a low total transferrin level. Storage iron is usually quite abundant. However, there is a decreased amount of iron in erythroblasts—this indicates a defect in the transfer of reticuloendothelial iron to immature red blood cells.

Board Testing Point: Understand the mechanisms involved with anemia of chronic disease.

358. Answer: C

Answer: Hemolysis is commonly induced by infection.
Viruses or bacterial infection are most common, and they induce an environmental oxidant stress. Drugs such as dapsone, sulfonamides, antimalarial agents, and vitamin K can also trigger hemolysis. The gene for G6PD is on the X chromosome; therefore, it is a sex-linked trait. Men are more commonly involved than women. The Mediterranean variant is more severe than the A type, which is found in the majority of African-Americans. The Heinz bodies can be seen only with special supravital stains. G6PD levels decrease as the red cell ages. So, during an acute episode of hemolysis, it is a bad time to check for the deficiency since a false-negative test will be seen—because the newer cells being made during hemolysis will have higher levels of G6PD than older cells.

Board Testing Point: Recognize the clinical features of G6PD deficiency.

359. Answer: B

Answer: Normochromic, normocytic red blood cells.
You would expect a very low reticulocyte count, not an elevated one. The bone marrow examination in pure red cell aplasia contrasts with aplastic anemia in that you expect to find a normocellular or hypercellular marrow in patients with pure red cell aplasia. Ferrokinetic studies would show a reduced iron turnover. Erythropoietin levels would be elevated in red cell aplasia.

Board Testing Point: Recognize the clinical characteristics seen in a pure red cell aplasia.

360. Answer: D

Answer: Check Factor VII level.
The finding of a prolonged PT and a normal PTT suggests a defect in the extrinsic coagulation cascade. Factor VII deficiency is **rare** and is autosomal recessive; however, looking at the choices, this is the best test to order.

Factor VIII deficiency, as well as the presence of coagulation factor inhibitors (Factor VIII inhibitor is the most common), would prolong the PTT. An α_2-antiplasmin deficiency results in a bleeding disorder with accelerated clot lysis; the PT and PTT are normal in these patients.

Board Testing Point: Understand how to interpret PT and PTT values and know that an isolated elevated PT is associated with Factor VII deficiency or inhibition.

361. Answer: A

Answer: Factor XII deficiency.
Platelet deficiency will result in normal PT and PTT, except bleeding time will be abnormal. von Willebrand's will result in normal PT and PTT, but an abnormally prolonged bleeding time with normal platelet aggregation. Factor VII deficiency will result in abnormal prolongation of the PT, but a normal PTT. Glanzmann thrombasthenia will result in a normal PT and PTT, but an abnormal bleeding time, as well as abnormal platelet aggregation.

Board Testing Point: Recognize that Factor XII deficiency does not usually result in a bleeding diathesis.

362. Answer: D

Answer: Patients lack glycoprotein Ib.
Patients have severely decreased platelet adhesion because of the lack of glycoprotein 1b. The platelets cannot bind to von Willebrand factor. They also have deficiency of glycoproteins V and IX. They usually have a modestly low platelet count also. It is an autosomal recessive disease.

Board Testing Point: Know the defect in Bernard-Soulier syndrome.

363. Answer: B

Answer: It is due to a deficiency of platelet integrin alpha IIb beta 3.
This is an autosomal recessive disorder, but it can also be acquired with acquisition of allo- or auto-antibodies to platelet integrin alpha IIb beta 3 (formerly glycoprotein IIb-IIIa complex). The lack of this glycoprotein complex does **not** permit fibrinogen to cross-connect, resulting in severe bleeding. Platelet counts are usually normal in this disease.

Board Testing Point: Know the defect responsible for Glanzmann thrombasthenia.

364. Answer: E

Answer: Iron deficiency anemia.
The patient has the classic symptoms and findings of iron deficiency anemia. Her history of menorrhagia is common and frequently results in iron deficiency anemia in younger women. At her age, the other possible diagnoses listed are very unlikely.

Board Testing Point: Recognize the clinical features of iron deficiency anemia.

365. Answer: E

Answer: Alcoholism.
By definition he has a macrocytic anemia. Luckily, only a few things will do this: alcoholism (due to interference with folic acid metabolism), B_{12} deficiency, myelodysplastic syndrome, etc. Vitamin B_{12} deficiency is relatively rare and with his current diet is unlikely to develop. Myelodysplastic syndrome occurs in his age group, but is less common, and we see evidence of liver disease with the presence of target cells, as well as the mildly elevated transaminases. Iron deficiency anemia would not give this picture.

Board Testing Point: Recognize that alcoholism is one of the most common causes of macrocytosis in the United States.

366. Answer: C

Answer: Hairy cell leukemia.
Note that hairy cell leukemia is a neoplasm of mature B-lymphocytes, typically presenting with pancytopenia, splenomegaly, and a dry bone marrow aspirate. Patients with hairy cell are prone to infections with unusual organisms like atypical mycobacteria. Bone marrow findings can include "fried egg" appearance in that cells appear to be separated from each other due to the "projections and fixation artifacts" generated by the hairy cells. It is easily treated and responds well to chemotherapy. Pancytopenia with a dry tap goes against CLL and myeloma. Normal RBC morphology goes against myelofibrosis. The WBC and differential go against CML.

Board Testing Point: Recognize the clinical and laboratory features of hairy cell leukemia.

367. Answer: D

Answer: Factor XIII deficiency.
This disorder may be inherited or acquired and frequently causes severe bleeding problems. In this disorder, the bleeding time, PT, and PTT are all normal! The screening test for Factor XIII deficiency is checking a "clot solubility in urea assay." It is very rare but is most common in individuals from Iran (due to increased consanguinity).

People with Factor XII and prekallikrein deficiency also have prolongation of PTT but do not have problems with surgery. Normal bleeding time excludes thrombasthenia, an inherited disorder of platelet aggregation. Protein S is a vitamin K-dependent plasma protein and a cofactor for expression of the anticoagulant activity of activated protein C.

Board Testing Point: Recognize the clinical and laboratory features of Factor XIII deficiency.

368. Answer: E

Answer: Protamine sulfate.
Protamine sulfate is **inappropriate**. She has warfarin-induced skin necrosis due to protein C deficiency. She probably has acquired the disease from her liver dysfunction. The cutaneous vessels thrombosed when warfarin was added without heparin. Since protein C has a short half-life, warfarin inactivates this protein before any of the other clotting factors. This can lead to a temporary procoagulant state that is exacerbated in a patient who is already deficient in protein C. If immediate intervention is not begun, the lesion will spread and she will develop skin necrosis. Treatment is to stop warfarin and start heparin. You also should administer vitamin K to counteract any further effect warfarin may be having. If all this fails, then give protein C concentrate or protein C-containing products, such as fresh frozen plasma. Protamine counteracts heparin and is contraindicated.

Board Testing Point: Recognize warfarin-induced skin necrosis and know which agents may be used in therapy.

369. Answer: D

Answer: B_{12} deficiency due to omeprazole use.
This patient has Zollinger-Ellison syndrome, which is managed through the use of high-dose proton pump inhibitors. High doses of proton pump inhibitors can decrease absorption of vitamin B_{12}. Oral B_{12} absorption is reduced by 90% in volunteers taking 40 mg of omeprazole.

Board Testing Point: Recognize that proton pump inhibitors at high dose for a prolonged period of time can inhibit absorption of vitamin B_{12}.

370. Answer: C

Answer: Chronic myelogenous leukemia (CML).
The "Philadelphia chromosome" is seen in all CML and some cases of acute lymphoblastic leukemia (Ph + ALL). Tyrosine kinase inhibitors (TKI) like imatinib/dasatinib and nilotinib can be used to target this chromosomal abnormality. In Ph + ALL, TKIs are used in combination with aggressive chemotherapy regimens.

Board Testing Point: Recognize the association of the Philadelphia chromosome t(9,22) with chronic myelogenous leukemia.

371. Answer: A

Answer: Hereditary spherocytosis.
The clues here are the splenomegaly at age 20, the elevated MCHC, increased osmotic fragility, and the decreased red cell survival. The history of gallstones in relatives at early ages is also common in this disease. It is quite common and occurs in 1/5,000 in northern Europeans.

Board Testing Point: Recognize the clinical features of hereditary spherocytosis.

372. Answer: D

Answer: A cutaneous vasculitis may also appear in this condition.
The patient has hairy cell leukemia. It frequently can be difficult to distinguish from polyarteritis. Neutropenia is quite common, as well as pancytopenia. The disease is associated with defects in both humoral and cellular immunity and will respond to alpha-interferon. Splenectomy will not be curative, since it will not affect the marrow. The cytoplasmic projections are classic for this disease process.

Board Testing Point: Recognize the clinical features of hairy cell leukemia.

373. Answer: B

Answer: 1:1 mix of patient and normal to measure the PTT.
This patient has a prolonged PTT leading to bleeding. This is not a LAC or anticardiolipin antibody, because the patient is bleeding and these syndromes should cause clotting. The next step in the evaluation should be a 1:1 mix of patient and normal to evaluate for correction of the PTT. The PTT corrects initially but then prolongs with incubation, which is indicative of an inhibitor that is most commonly affecting Factor VIII—but could be any of the other factors in the intrinsic pathway.

Board Testing Point: Understand how to work up a patient with an elevated PTT to determine if an inhibitor is present.

ONCOLOGY

374. Answer: B

Answer: Acute myelogenous leukemia (AML).
AML is unusual in that lymphadenopathy is **not** common. Splenomegaly is also **not** common in AML.

Board Testing Point: Recognize that AML does not usually have lymphadenopathy or splenomegaly.

---

375. Answer: B

Answer: Acute myelogenous leukemia.
She has gingival hyperplasia! She also doesn't have an enlarged spleen. The gingival hyperplasia is seen in nearly 1/2 of patients with monocytic AML (M5). The other possible etiologies listed are unlikely to do this.

Board Testing Point: Recognize the clinical features associated with acute myelogenous leukemia (AML).

---

376. Answer: D

Answer: Neurotoxicity.
These patients can develop a peripheral neuropathy.

Board Testing Point: Know that use of vincristine is associated with peripheral neuropathy.

---

377. Answer: C

Answer: On immunophenotyping, CD11c marker is likely to be present.
Bone marrow aspirate in hairy cell leukemia is usually **dry** despite the fact that you have a **hypercellular** bone marrow on biopsy. This is due to increased reticulin. 2-CdA will induce a complete remission in 85–90% of patients! Hairy cell leukemia is one of the B-cell leukemias, like CLL. It comprises only about 2% of leukemias, but make sure you can recognize a "hairy" cell on smear.

Board Testing Point: Recognize that hairy cell leukemia is associated with the CD11c marker.

---

378. Answer: C

Answer: This is likely a side effect of tamoxifen; venlafaxine may be beneficial.
Tamoxifen is the drug of choice in pre- and perimenopausal women with ER/PR-positive breast cancer for adjuvant hormonal therapy; however, it is associated with risk of thromboembolic disease and causes hot flashes. The most likely explanation for her symptoms is hot flashes. SSRIs/SNRIs can improve the symptoms of hot flashes, but you can use only certain ones! Tamoxifen is converted to its active metabolites (endoxifen) by CYP2D6. Many SSRIs and SNRIs inhibit this enzyme and reduce the efficacy of tamoxifen.
The SSRIs/SNRIs that either do not inhibit CYP2D6 or do so minimally are:

- SSRIs: citalopram (Celexa®) and escitalopram (Lexipro®)
- SNRIs: venlafaxine (Effexor®) and desvenlafaxime (Pristiq®)

It is unlikely that this is due to recurrent thromboembolic disease, pericardial effusion, or brain metastasis because the patient has rapid clinical improvement and the symptoms could be called transient. Also, this is favorable early stage breast cancer that would usually not develop metastasis.

Board Testing Point: Know the side effects of tamoxifen and the treatment of these side effects. Understand that some of these treatments are contraindicated because they interfere with the conversion of tamoxifen to its active metabolite by interfering with CYP2D6.

379. Answer: A

Answer: Urgent MRI if diagnosis confirmed, then IV dexamethasone, followed by radiation oncology consult.
With leg weakness, point tenderness, and possible incontinence, the main concern is that of spinal cord compression due to vertebral body metastasis. While the spinal cord ends between L1 and L2, the compression of the cauda equina can also cause lower extremity weakness along with back pain and sensory abnormalities in the lower extremities, with saddle anesthesia of the back. For circumferential and single level compression, one can consider neurosurgical intervention. However, for extensive disease or poor performance status or radiosensitive tumors like small cell lung cancer, radiotherapy, along with steroids, would be the urgent treatment needed for this patient. The clinical picture, especially with point tenderness, goes against options of paraneoplastic myelopathy, disease progression, or brain metastasis.

Board Testing Point: Know how to recognize and manage cord compression, an oncological emergency.

380. Answer: A

Answer: Remove the central venous catheter and start empiric broad-spectrum antibiotics, as well as either liposomal amphotericin B or caspofungin.
In this severely neutropenic woman, and considering her overwhelmingly immunocompromised state from her recent transplant and medications, all bacterial etiologies as well as severe fungemias must be considered, particularly with *Candida* species. Therefore, it is reasonable to start broad-spectrum antibiotics as well as antifungal therapy (either liposomal amphotericin B or caspofungin) initially. The line must be removed at any sign of infection, particularly if fungal infection is suspected as it is in this woman.

Board Testing Point: Know the empiric therapy for a patient with severe neutropenia status post bone marrow transplant.

381. Answer: B

Answer: Change in the color of the lesion warrants further workup for potential malignancy.
One of the characteristics that distinguishes a superficial spreading malignant melanoma from a normal mole is a change in the color of the lesion. Another warning sign is if the border becomes irregular. Usually, the first change noted is a "darkening" in color or a change in the borders of the lesion. Excisional biopsy should be done promptly because early diagnosis and excision reduce mortality.

Board Testing Point: Recognize the clinical features that would warrant a workup of a potential malignant skin lesion.

382. Answer: D

Answer: Endoscopic visualization of the nasopharynx and larynx, and integrated PET-CT scan.
A firm neck mass in a smoker and heavy drinker is always suspicious for squamous cell carcinoma of the head and neck. The finding of squamous cell carcinoma on the biopsy warrants an aggressive search for a primary lesion in the head and neck region and, therefore, the multiple endoscopies are indicated. Integrated PET-CT scan is superior to CT, MRI, and PET scanning alone and will help determine primary tumor invasion of specific anatomic sites. Once a primary is determined and the extent of the disease is assessed, the decision on therapy can be made. Standard therapy for primary head and neck squamous cell carcinoma with lymph node metastasis is radiation therapy, surgery, or both. Adjuvant chemotherapy is being investigated to reduce tumor load before surgery or radiation.

Board Testing Point: Understand the staging and workup of a squamous cell carcinoma neck mass.

383. Answer: A

Answer: Huntington disease.
Huntington disease is **not** associated with development of malignancy.

Fanconi anemia is associated with cytogenetic abnormalities and has an increased risk of cancer. Approximately 10% of patients with neurofibromatosis develop sarcomatous changes. Ataxia-telangiectasia is associated with lymphoma. Familial polyposis coli predisposes to colon cancer in all patients with this disorder.

Board Testing Point: Recognize that many hereditary disorders are associated with later development of malignancy.

384. Answer: C

Answer: Anthracycline agents suppress bone marrow stem cells to a greater degree than they do more "committed" hematopoietic cells.
This is a false statement. The anthracycline agents generally suppress the more "committed" cells to a greater degree than the stem cell lines. The other statements are correct. Cisplatin can induce N/V, and it does cause large renal loses of potassium and magnesium that in turn leads to hypocalcemia. Vincristine is a relatively mild myelosuppressive agent and can be used in periods of low white blood cell counts. And melphalan has been associated with secondary leukemias.

Board Testing Point: Recognize toxic effects of chemotherapeutic agents.

385. Answer: E

Answer: Administer leuprolide.
GnRH agonist therapy is at least as effective as orchiectomy and will spare him surgery as well as the complications of surgery. Knowing that he had poorly differentiated disease at initial diagnosis and now with the findings of bone lesions in his ribs and pelvis, biopsy is not necessary. Prostate cancer is not very responsive to chemotherapy such as cisplatin.

Board Testing Point: Recognize that GnRH agonist therapy is the best initial therapy for metastatic prostate cancer.

386. Answer: B

Answer: Bone scan to show increased uptake.
A bone scan would not be helpful for identifying multiple myeloma. Myeloma causes osteolytic lesions, not osteoblastic lesions. Remember: A bone scan can pick up only osteoblastic lesions. The skeletal survey would be very helpful in determining extent of disease, as would the β_2-microglobulin. Renal involvement is quite common with multiple myeloma, and determination of 24-hour urine protein excretion can be helpful in determining prognosis. Serum protein electrophoresis is also helpful in diagnosis.

Board Testing Point: Recognize that a bone scan will not be helpful in determining location of bony lesions in multiple myeloma.

387. Answer: B

Answer: Ovarian cancer of germ cell lineage.
Most ovarian cancers are of epithelial cell lineage; however, she had evidence of hormonal abnormalities with the hirsutism, deepening voice, and clitorimegaly. All of these findings are consistent with virilization and androgen production. These ovarian germ cell tumors can be treated similarly to testicular carcinoma in men and respond to therapy with cisplatin and etoposide.

Board Testing Point: Recognize the clinical features of an ovarian cancer with germ cell lineage.

388. Answer: E

Answer: Mantle cell lymphoma (a type of mature B cell non-Hodgkin lymphoma).
The key with this lymphoma is the immunophenotypical characteristics: The cells express B-cell antigens such as CD19 and CD20 as well as the nominal T-cell antigen CD5. This B-cell lymphoma is one of the only B-cell lymphomas to express this antigen! Chronic lymphocytic leukemia will do it too! Additionally, the t(11;14) translocation is nearly always associated with mantle cell lymphoma! What does the t(11;14) translocation do? It brings cyclin D_1 under the influence of immunoglobulin heavy chain promoters and leads to cyclin D_1 overexpression. But remember: CD19, CD20, and CD5 positivity and t(11;14) translocation mean mantle cell lymphoma!!

Board Testing Point: Recognize the clinical and immunophenotypical characteristics of mantle cell lymphoma (a type of mature-B cell non-Hodgkin lymphoma).

389. Answer: A

Answer: He has entered an accelerated or blastic phase.
The Philadelphia chromosome is the diagnostic "hallmark" of chronic myeloid leukemia. Remember that it involves the translocation between chromosome 22 and chromosome 9. Patients with CML usually have a chronic benign phase for 3–4 years. The most commonly observed cytogenetic event to signify an accelerated or blast phase is duplication of the Philadelphia chromosome!

Board Testing Point: Recognize the clinical significance of a duplicated Philadelphia chromosome in a patient with CML.

390. Answer: C

Answer: Ultrasound of the testicle.
A testicular mass in a young man must be further evaluated. Usually, an ultrasound will help differentiate a solid mass from a cyst or epididymitis. Once a malignancy is suspected (solid mass), then pre-surgical evaluation of tumor markers with AFP and beta hCG is needed followed by removal of the mass with an inguinal approach. With an elevated AFP, the tumor is definitely **not** a pure seminoma, despite the pathology report, and should be treated as a nonseminoma.

Board Testing Point: Understand the initial workup of a testicular mass.

391. Answer: D

Answer: Early-onset coronary artery disease.
Within months of mantle radiation therapy, about 15% of patients develop **lower** extremity paresthesia upon flexion of the neck, also known as Lhermitte sign. Radiation pneumonitis is also a concern in a small percentage of patients (< 5%). Other complications of mantle radiation include pericardial effusion, myocardial injury, and an increased risk of coronary artery disease. Hypothyroidism occurs in over 80% of patients! Breast cancer and lung cancer are increased in incidence, as well as stomach, skin, and soft tissue sarcomas. Acute leukemias are rare in patients not treated with chemotherapy agents.

Board Testing Point: Recognize the clinical complications of mantle radiation therapy.

392. Answer: A

Answer: Colposcopy.
Cervical cancer mortality is so preventable because it is easily revealed by the Pap smear; however, it's only a screening test. If the Pap returns with low-grade squamous intraepithelial lesion (or high-grade), a colposcopy with punch biopsy is required for diagnosis of CIN or invasive carcinoma. If the biopsy then shows CIN I (slight dysplasia), this may resolve and does not require treatment. A follow-up is recommended with a repeat Pap smear in 4–6 months. CIN II and III (moderate and severe dysplasia) are treated with ablative therapy, either cryotherapy or laser. If the punch biopsy returns showing invasive carcinoma, staging is done, and the patient is treated with hysterectomy or radiation, or both. If the biopsy did not make the stage of the premalignancy clear, then conization is indicated.

Board Testing Point: Recognize that colposcopy is generally the next procedure after finding any abnormality on a Pap smear.

393. Answer: B

Answer: Serous or mucinous epithelial cancer.
The diagnosis, considering the patient's age, her *BRCA1*-associated risk, and elevated CA-125, is almost certainly ovarian cancer. Half of all ovarian cancer patients are over age 65, and there is a 40% lifetime risk of ovarian cancer associated with the presence of *BRCA1* (compared to 1.5% risk in the female population overall.) The *BRCA1* gene, found in 5% of women, is also associated with a 50 to 80% lifetime risk of developing breast cancer. The CA-125 is commonly increased in ovarian cancer, and should be obtained in any patient suspected of having this disease. Serous and mucinous epithelial carcinomas are by far the most common ovarian cancers. (85% of ovarian cancer is epithelial cell, 1/2 of these serous, and 1/4 mucinous.) Germ cell cancers, including choriocarcinoma, usually occur in younger patients, and can elevate both alpha-fetoprotein and hCG. These 2 levels are not increased in epithelial carcinoma. Clear cell carcinoma, another epithelial cell type, is uncommon.

Board Testing Point: Be familiar with the different types of ovarian cancer and recognize that serous and mucinous epithelial carcinomas are the most common.

394. Answer: B

Answer: Chemotherapy, radiotherapy, and tamoxifen.
Although this is a small tumor, less than a centimeter, the presence of a positive axillary node means that she should receive adjuvant therapy as if it were large. Because the tumor was found to be HR+, both chemotherapy and tamoxifen are recommended. All lumpectomies include node dissection and should be followed with radiotherapy in order to be "the equivalent" of a mastectomy. Tamoxifen (or an aromatase inhibitor) as a sole agent can be used only if the patient is postmenopausal, a modified radical mastectomy is done, no positive nodes are found, and the tumor is HR+.

Understand that breast cancer therapy is difficult and controversial. Know that radiotherapy goes with lumpectomy; HR+ tumors require hormonal therapy; and adjuvant chemotherapy is recommended for most node-positive, large tumors, or advanced tumors.

Board Testing Point: Recognize common features/recommendations for breast cancer therapy that are noncontroversial.

395. Answer: B

Answer: Seminoma.
Seminomas comprise 60% of germ cell tumors, and nonseminomas the remaining 40%. Germ cell tumors comprise 95% of all testicular tumors. Sertoli cell cancer is uncommon. Torsion is an acute process accompanied by intense pain and tenderness. Hydroceles are cystic, not solid or firm.

Board Testing Point: Recognize that seminomas are the most common testicular tumors.

396. Answer: A

Answer: Acute myelogenous leukemia (AML).
All of the other malignancies will usually result in splenomegaly. This can be helpful when trying to differentiate AML from the other entities.

Board Testing Point: Recognize that splenomegaly is uncommon in acute myelogenous leukemia.

397. Answer: D

Answer: Proceed with combination chemotherapy without laparotomy.
This patient has Stage IIIB Hodgkin disease. Further workup is not needed since the CT scan and PET scan indicated disease on both sides of the diaphragm. Additionally, he has "B" symptoms with night sweats. Treatment should proceed with combination chemotherapy. Further surgery or workup is not indicated at this time.

Board Testing Point: Recognize that Stage IIIB Hodgkin disease requires treatment with combination chemotherapy.

398. Answer: A

Answer: > 75% are B-cell lymphomas.
Know that most non-Hodgkin lymphomas are B-cell type. Follicular lymphomas are usually quite **indolent**. Burkitt lymphoma is a type of non-Hodgkin lymphoma, and the African form is associated with Epstein-Barr virus infection.

Board Testing Point: Know that most non-Hodgkin lymphomas are of B-cell origin.

399. Answer: E

Answer: The lytic lesions on plain films would <u>not</u> "light up" on the bone scan.
This patient most likely has multiple myeloma. Multiple myeloma cells produce osteoclast activating factor, which induces the osteoclast to form lytic bone lesions **without** new bone formation. New bone formation is required for "lighting up" on the bone scan. It is unlikely that this patient would have osteomyelitis because of his multiple myeloma. Neither renal failure nor rouleaux formation would be contraindications for bone scan.

Board Testing Point: Recognize that in multiple myeloma a bone scan would not show increased activity.

400. Answer: C

Answer: Vigorous hydration with normal saline to maintain urine output at 100–150 cc/hour followed by zoledronic acid.
The best treatment is to hydrate the patient aggressively. Until recently, many also recommended the use of furosemide to help with calcium excretion; however, this has fallen out of favor because of the availability of bisphosphonates and calcitonin, as well as the increased risk of electrolyte abnormalities associated with furosemide use. Zoledronic acid will not work acutely but will begin to work in the first 24 hours to help provide prolonged response. A volume expander like normal saline is required and not 1/4 normal saline, which is comparable to free water.

Board Testing Point: Recommend treatment for hypercalcemia in a patient with cancer.

401. Answer: B

Answer: If the genital warts are due to human papillomavirus type 16 or 18.
These HPV types are thought to express an E7 protein that binds to the retinoblastoma protein, inactivating the retinoblastoma tumor-suppressor gene. Types 31 and 35 have also been implicated.

Board Testing Point: Know that HPV types 16 and 18 have increased risk of cervical cancer.

402. Answer: C

Answer: Combination of pelvic irradiation and chemotherapy.
She has regional lymph node involvement without metastasis, Dukes C, so chemotherapy is indicated. She has rectal carcinoma too, so radiation therapy is helpful in this context.

Board Testing Point: Know the therapy for Dukes C colon cancer with rectal carcinoma.

403. Answer: B

Answer: Bone scan.
This is the first staging test done in the workup of prostate cancers that are at higher risk (the PSA of ≥ 20 puts him at higher risk). If abnormalities are found on the bone scan, you then proceed to do plain-film x-rays of the areas to exclude other possible causes. Then you would do surgical staging with removal and examination of the surrounding nodes (often done with prostatectomy). Recent data show that those at lower risk (T2 or lower, Gleason Score < 6, and PSA < 10) do not necessarily require bone scan for staging.

Board Testing Point: Know that high-risk prostate cancer workup usually includes bone scan.

404. Answer: A

Answer: 95%.
With a seminoma confined to the testes (Stage I), there is a 95% survival rate with radiation therapy. This is one of the most curable types of cancer, especially if recognized and treated early.

Board Testing Point: Recognize that testicular cancer is highly curable if diagnosed at an early stage.

405. Answer: E

Answer: Modified radical mastectomy with chemotherapy and tamoxifen.
The lesion is > 4 cm; therefore, she should get a modified radical mastectomy, and most would give chemotherapy because of the size of the tumor. She is postmenopausal, so you must look at her hormone receptor (HR) status to determine what to do next. If it is HR-positive, she gets tamoxifen. If it is HR-negative, she gets only chemotherapy.

Board Testing Point: Know that large tumors of the breast require modified radical mastectomy, adjuvant chemotherapy, and, if HR+, hormonal therapy.

406. Answer: B

Answer: Modified radical mastectomy with chemotherapy and tamoxifen for 5 years.
The lesion is > 4 cm; therefore, she should get a modified radical mastectomy. She is premenopausal, so she should also get chemotherapy (note that if she was postmenopausal the tumor size would persuade most to also give chemotherapy). Finally, you need to know the hormonal status to determine if she should get tamoxifen. If it is positive, she gets tamoxifen. If it is negative, she gets only chemotherapy and no tamoxifen.

Board Testing Point: Know therapy for breast cancer.

407. Answer: E

Answer: Oral contraceptive use.
Oral contraceptive use is not associated with increased risk of ovarian cancer and actually will decrease risk. *BRCA1* (17q21) is associated with a 40% lifetime risk of developing ovarian cancer and accounts for most patients with familial ovarian cancer. *BRCA2* (13q12-13) is associated with a 10–20% risk of ovarian cancer. Nulliparity and a positive family history also both increase risk but to a lesser extent.

Board Testing Point: Recognize risk factors for ovarian cancer.

408. Answer: A

Answer: Multiple myeloma.
This elderly patient has bone pain, hypercalcemia, and anemia. His x-ray shows osteoporosis, and he has a negative bone scan. The best fit for a diagnosis would be multiple myeloma. Myeloma can cause diffuse osteoporosis as well as anemia and hypercalcemia. An important pearl about myeloma is that bone lesions do not show up on bone scan. Metastatic prostate or lung cancer would likely show up on bone scan. Prolonged steroid use and avascular necrosis would not cause hypercalcemia and anemia.

Board Testing Point: Recognize the clinical features of multiple myeloma.

409. Answer: A

Answer: Breast cancer.
Unfortunately, even with physical examination of the breast combined with mammogram, a good number of breast cancers will be undiagnosed before they disseminate.

Board Testing Point: Recognize that breast cancer may disseminate or be advanced even without a palpable breast mass.

410. Answer: B

Answer: Metastatic germ cell tumor of the testis.
The findings of endocrine abnormalities (gynecomastia) at initial presentation support a germ cell tumor. So too does the now enlarged testis, which may not have been present at the time of initial diagnosis. Pulmonary metastases with germ cell tumor of the testis is common.

Board Testing Point: Recognize the association of gynecomastia with a germ cell tumor.

411. Answer: E

Answer: Doxorubicin (Adriamycin®, Rubex®).
It is **not** associated with peripheral neuropathy. Know that doxorubicin's main concern is cardiac abnormalities.

Board Testing Point: Know the side effects of common chemotherapeutic agents.

412. Answer: D

Answer: Small cell lung cancer.
Small cell carcinoma of the lung is most closely associated with SIADH. Remember, "small cells" do a lot of stuff, including SIADH, ectopic ACTH production, and Eaton-Lambert (myasthenic) syndrome.

Board Testing Point: Recognize that SIADH is associated with small cell carcinoma of the lung.

413. Answer: A

Answer: Ovarian cancer.
This is pretty straightforward. Just memorize it. Also, you may have noticed this topic was mentioned in another question, but use of oral contraceptives and their risks of cancers come up quite often on the exam.

Board Testing Point: Know that oral contraceptives reduce risk of ovarian cancer.

414. Answer: C

Answer: Urgent medical oncology consult for chemotherapy.
Mediastinal germ cell tumors, both seminoma and non-seminoma, respond well to chemotherapy. It is very important to get biopsy serum markers beta hCG, AFP, and LDH prior to therapy as a baseline. In the case of chemo-sensitive tumors like small cell lung cancer, nonseminomatous germ cell tumor in solid tumors, and lymphoma in hematological malignancies, SVC syndrome is treated initially with chemotherapy rather than surgical excision, stent, or radiation. (Even in the case of seminoma, which is very radiosensitive, the general rule of thumb would be chemotherapy first.) The caveat: If this is teratoma, then it does not respond well to chemotherapy and needs to be excised.

Use of steroids in SVC syndrome is controversial; however, it can help if the tumor is lymphoma. A patient with bulky chemo-sensitive mediastinal tumors should be monitored for tumor lysis syndrome upon initiation of therapy.

Board Testing Point: Know how to manage oncological urgency SVC syndrome in relation to type of tumor.

415. Answer: D

Answer: Blood transfusion.
The patient's neutropenia is unlikely to be the cause of his symptoms. Also, he does not appear infected, he is afebrile, and his symptoms have been more progressive than acute. His symptoms seem mainly related to anemia; however, while erythroid-stimulating agents like erythropoietin and darbepoetin can be used to improve the symptoms related to anemia, they increase cancer-related death due to cancer progression. Hence, they should not be used in the adjuvant setting. Even in the metastatic setting, health care providers need to undergo special training to prescribe these to be able to discuss the risks and benefits of the cancer progression. Iron therapy is unlikely to help; hence, blood transfusion to treat symptoms of anemia is the best option.

Board Testing Point: Awareness of risk of erythroid-stimulating agents in increasing cancer-related mortality in certain solid tumors and their avoidance.

416. Answer: A

Answer: High potassium (K), high phosphorus (P), low calcium (Ca), and high uric acid (UA).
When tumor cells break down by auto tumor lysis or due to therapy, they release their intracellular contents into the blood, which causes electrolyte abnormalities of hyperkalemia, hypercalcemia, and hyperuricemia. Typically, it is associated with hypocalcemia because calcium is bound by phosphorus, leading to calcium phosphate crystal deposits in the kidney, ultimately leading to renal failure and multiorgan failure. Adequate prophylaxis, immediate recognition, and treatment with dialysis and rasburicase can be lifesaving.

Board Testing Point: Be able to recognize and manage of tumor lysis syndrome as an oncological emergency.

417. Answer: B

Answer: A screening breast MRI now.
Screening breast mammogram is recommended for most women who are ≥ 50 years of age. However, breast MRI is recommended for screening in patients with 1st degree relatives with *BRCA1* or *BRCA2*; women with lifetime risk of breast cancer of ≥ 20–25%; patients who had radiation to the chest between ages 10 and 30 years; and carriers of, or 1st degree relatives with, the TP53 (Li Fraumeni syndrome), *PTEN* mutation (Cowden syndrome), or hereditary diffuse gastric cancer syndrome. Breast ultrasound is not recommended for screening in any population; it is used more as a tool to follow up lesions on mammogram.

Board Testing Point: Understand the indications for different imaging modalities for breast cancer screening.

418. Answer: D

Answer: Hold zoledronic acid and refer the patient back to oral surgery.
This is likely osteonecrosis of the jaw (ONJ) due to dental procedure done in the setting of prolonged bisphosphonate use; this practice should be avoided. Dental procedures and evaluation should be completed prior to bisphosphonate use in the nonemergent setting. Symptoms include localized pain, swelling and inflammation of the gums, and loosening of teeth. It is usually identified by the appearance of exposed bone in the oral cavity. Once ONJ occurs, it is advisable not to use bisphosphonates again. Metastases usually do not occur in the jaw bone.

Board Testing Point: Be able to recognize and manage complications of bisphosphonates, which are widely used in oncological disease.

NEUROLOGY

419. Answer: E

Answer: No imaging.
This patient has typical symptoms of migraine headaches. She is at a common age (22) for the onset of migraines. Migraines are more common in women. Aura occurs in about 25% of cases. The quality standards subcommittee of the American Academy of Neurology does not recommend the use of CNS imaging in adult patients with recurrent headaches typical of migraine, without focal neurologic signs or symptoms.

Board Testing Point: Know that imaging is not required in the workup of classic migraine.

420. Answer: A

Answer: Dix-Hallpike maneuver.
This patient has very brief episodes of vertigo, which usually occur when he has a sudden change of position such as rolling over in bed. This is the classic description of benign positional vertigo. This diagnosis is confirmed clinically with the Dix-Hallpike maneuver.

You have the patient sit on the examination table with legs extended. You turn their head 30° to 45° toward one side and then help the patient quickly lie back so their head hangs over the end of the table. You then watch their eyes for involuntary eye movements (nystagmus). After they sit upright for a few minutes to recover from the vertigo, the procedure is repeated with their head turned in the opposite direction. There is no specific testing such as an audiogram ENG or MRI that would make this diagnosis. Additionally, he has no complaints of hearing loss.

Board Testing Point: Recognize the clinical syndrome associated with benign positional vertigo and know that the Dix-Hallpike maneuver is the best method to diagnose.

421. Answer: A

Answer: Subarachnoid hemorrhage.
The sequence of events is critical to the diagnosis. The headache was sudden: "Thunder-clap" and "Worst headache of my life" are common descriptors. It is not unusual for a person to lose consciousness with a subarachnoid bleed. Often, they appear better following this, and then worsen. The sign that shows meningeal irritation is meningismus. A low-grade fever is common. A stroke would not cause meningismus. Herpes is usually slower in onset, and associated with a high fever. Often, herpes causes changes in mentation prior to other symptoms. Abscesses and tumors are more likely to cause focal neurological deficits.

Board Testing Point: Recognize the clinical features of subarachnoid hemorrhage.

422. Answer: A

Answer: CT scan without contrast.
This patient has symptoms consistent with acute subarachnoid hemorrhage. He is at the average age (45) for this to occur, has sudden onset of a severe headache, and no prior history of severe headaches. The neck stiffness is due to meningeal irritation from blood. Blood in the subarachnoid space shows up very well on CT scan, and contrast is **not** needed. Acute bleeds are better imaged by non-contrast CT scan than with MRIs. The CT scan is a preferable first option over a lumbar puncture, because if the CT is positive, an LP would not be necessary. The non-contrast CT has a sensitivity of about 95% in the first 24 hours of symptoms, the sensitivity drops to about 50% at day 7. If the CT is negative, then an LP should be done looking for xanthochromia, which occurs 6 hours after SAH and can last for up to 2–4 weeks.

Board Testing Point: Recognize the clinical features of subarachnoid hemorrhage and know that CT scan without contrast is the best screening tool.

---

423. Answer: D

Answer: Head MRI.
This 31-year-old woman has recurrent neurologic symptoms, with improvement between episodes. This history is suggestive of multiple sclerosis (MS). The most sensitive imaging procedure for MS is MRI. Although lesions can occur in the spinal cord, the brain is the best first imaging site. The brain MRI shows lesions in over 92% of patients with MS.

Board Testing Point: Recognize the clinical characteristics of multiple sclerosis and know that MRI is indicated for diagnosis.

---

424. Answer: E

Answer: Reaction to phenytoin.
This patient is having a reaction to phenytoin, creating pseudolymphoma syndrome. He has fever, elevated transaminases, and generalized lymphadenopathy. A negative RPR effectively rules out secondary syphilis. He has no exposure history to suggest hepatitis B or tularemia. Hodgkin disease is a possibility, but the involvement of the liver with diffuse lymphadenopathy would indicate advanced disease, which would be unlikely to occur so rapidly.

Board Testing Point: Recognize the pseudolymphoma syndrome associated with phenytoin use.

---

425. Answer: C

Answer: Stop tramadol.
This older patient is evaluated for seizure. You are given the information that he has a negative contrast head CT scan. This makes tumor as a cause very unlikely. He is on tramadol, a medication that has been associated with seizures. This medication should be stopped, and the patient should have further evaluation only if he has additional seizures off this medication. His presentation is not suggestive of an infectious process such as meningitis or encephalitis, thus an LP is not indicated. AEDs should not be started after a single likely provoked tramadol seizure.

Board Testing Point: Recognize that tramadol may cause seizures, especially in the elderly.

---

426. Answer: E

Answer: Oral contraceptive pills.
This patient has had headaches for 6 months. The most likely diagnosis is headache associated with oral contraceptive pills. She has a small risk for pseudotumor cerebri because she is obese. This diagnosis is excluded by the normal funduscopic because papilledema is a hallmark of this. There are no cutaneous features suggestive of tuberous sclerosis (ash leaf spot, adenoma sebaceum).

Board Testing Point: Recognize that oral contraceptive pills are a common cause of headache.

---

427. Answer: C

Answer: Gabapentin.
This elderly patient is suffering from postherpetic neuralgia. Because of his history of coronary artery disease and BPH, tricyclic antidepressants (amitriptyline and nortriptyline) would be contraindicated. In patients with BPH, tricyclics can cause acute urinary retention. There is a higher risk for arrhythmia in patients with CAD treated with tricyclics. Gabapentin is effective and well tolerated for the treatment of post-herpetic neuralgia. Narcotics can be used for treatment of post-herpetic neuralgia, but a long-acting narcotic like hydrocodone/oxycodone would not be the first option. Narcotics are more toxic in the elderly, and in this case could lead to urinary retention. The anti-seizure medications gabapentin and carbamazepine are effective for post-herpetic neuralgia. Phenytoin is not usually used because of toxicity and unproven efficacy.

Board Testing Point: Know that gabapentin is a good initial drug for post-herpetic neuralgia, especially compared to other agents that have multiple side effects.

---

428. Answer: D

Answer: Multiple sensory deficits.
This elderly patient notices disequilibrium when she walks. The key information is that her symptoms are improved when she touches a wall. She does not have vertigo symptoms. If she had orthostatic hypotension, her symptoms would not improve with touching a wall. Both benign positional vertigo and vestibular neuronitis have symptoms of vertigo, which this patient does not have. She is elderly, which is the population multiple sensory deficits are seen in. These patients may have visual, hearing, orthopedic, and neuropathy problems. The sum total of these sensory problems makes the patient feel unsteady. When sensory input from the hand (touching the wall) is included, she feels more stable.

Board Testing Point: Recognize the clinical symptoms of multiple sensory deficits causing disequilibrium.

---

429. Answer: A

Answer: Have the patient call 911 for emergency evaluation/transport to emergency department.
This patient has symptoms consistent with CO poisoning: headache, nausea, vomiting, diarrhea, and dyspnea. The key piece of clinical information is the improvement when he went outside to shovel snow. The appropriate management would be immediate removal from his home and immediate supportive care in an emergency department. Remember that the SPO_2 and PO_2 will be normal. Indications for hyperbaric oxygenation inculde coma, pregnancy, acidosis and a CO level above 30%. Hyperbaric oxygenation reduces the half life of CO from 300 mins (on room air) to 25–30 minutes on HBOT.

Board Testing Point: Recognize how subtle carbon monoxide poisoning can be.

430. Answer: B

Answer: Seizure (post-ictal).
When confronted with a question like this, narrow the list first. Stroke is unlikely because of his age and the lack of focal neurologic findings. Encephalitis is unlikely without a fever and elevated white count. Hyperglycemia is out. The routine labs are negative. Drug intoxication is possible, as is a seizure/post-ictal state. Of these choices, seizure wins over drug intoxication because of the lack of findings on examination (no papillary abnormalities).

Board Testing Point: Be able to differentiate quickly among seizure, stroke, encephalitis, and drug intoxications.

431. Answer: C

Answer: Toxicology.
Although several of the tests would probably be performed while the patient is in the emergency department, remember to look for **a single, best answer**. Given that there is no evidence of trauma, and no focal neurological deficits, the CT and skull x-ray are unlikely to help. The lack of meningeal signs eliminates diagnoses like encephalitis and subarachnoid hemorrhage, so the lumbar puncture is less likely to help. An ABG might help if carbon monoxide (CO) poisoning were suspected; however, we are told that his apartment was well ventilated. Also, CO poisoning occurs most often in older persons who use petroleum-burning space heaters in the winter. Although we see no evidence of drug intoxication on exam, toxicology would be very helpful in this situation.

Board Testing Point: Know the best test to perform on an unconscious, unresposponsive patient to narrow the differential.

432 Answer: C

Answer: Cluster headache.
The combination of a normal exam with these headache symptoms describes a cluster headache. For the exam, you must know the differences among each of the listed headaches. Cluster headaches are more common in males and respond to 100% oxygen.

Board Testing Point: Recognize the clinical features of cluster headache.

433. Answer: B

Answer: Abscess.
In this case, the gradually worsening headaches after an invasive procedure strongly suggest a post-operative abscess. The fever and focal neurological deficits confirm this. Remember, the triad of fever, focal deficits, and headache means **abscess**. Her pupils are normal and, with the focal findings, this excludes opiate intoxication.

Board Testing Point: Recognize the clinical features of a brain abscess.

---

434. Answer: D

Answer: Ménière disease.
The triad of episodic vertigo, hearing loss, and tinnitus makes this the most likely diagnosis. In benign positional vertigo, the person would not be expected to have hearing loss. Labyrinthitis and neuronitis are usually monophasic illnesses, likely due to a virus. Although stroke can cause vertigo, it is unlikely to be recurrent. In addition, stroke rarely causes vertigo by itself. The hearing loss in Ménière disease is usually progressive.

Board Testing Point: Recognize a classic presentation of Ménière disease.

---

435. Answer: A

Answer: Cerebellar infarct.
Infarct is most likely to explain the sudden onset of this constellation of signs and symptoms. Cerebellar infarct is very dangerous, and anyone with this diagnosis should be observed closely. Maximal swelling may occur up to 96 hours post infarction. As swelling occurs, there is a risk of compression of the brainstem. If the brainstem is at risk, surgery may be necessary as a life-saving procedure. Nystagmus and ataxia would not occur with BPV or Ménière disease.

Board Testing Point: Recognize the clinical features of a cerebellar infarct.

---

436. Answer: B

Answer: Multiple sclerosis.
The most likely diagnosis is multiple sclerosis (MS). The history of transient neurologic dysfunction (the blurred vision in college) strongly supports the diagnosis. The patient has an upper motor neuron disease (the increased reflexes and positive Babinski), so Cauda Equina syndrome and Guillain-Barré are not possible. The symptoms involve only the left side, so transverse myelitis, which would cause a paraparesis, is not possible. Stroke is unlikely because the patient is young, without risk factors for stroke, and the symptoms have gradually worsened for 10 days. She denies orthostatic hypotension.

Board Testing Point: Recognize the clinical features of multiple sclerosis.

---

437. Answer: B

Answer: Parkinson disease.
Since he is on no medications, he does not have a drug-induced Parkinsonism (not a choice here). Shy-Drager by definition includes severe orthostasis. Striatonigral degeneration looks like Parkinson's without the resting tremor. PSP includes loss of voluntary vertical gaze and axial rigidity (more than appendicular). PSP is also highly associated with dementia. Alzheimer's and Parkinson's can overlap. However, Alzheimer's does not begin with these symptoms, and is therefore very unlikely.

Board Testing Point: Describe the clinical manifestations of Parkinson disease.

438. Answer: E

Answer: Tensilon® test (if available); if not available, then acetylcholine receptor antibodies (AChR-Ab).
This patient has a characteristic presentation of myasthenia gravis. The age of onset is between the 2nd and 4th decades of life. Myasthenia is due to circulating polyclonal IgG autoantibodies (produced by B-lymphocytes) to the acetylcholine receptor. It is characterized by weakness that worsens with physical activity. In about 40% of cases, the presenting complaint is diplopia. Other common symptoms include dysarthria, dysphagia, and decreased range of facial movements. Limb and neck weakness is common. It is uncommon for the limbs to be affected without other symptoms. Medications such as D-penicillamine (once used to treat rheumatoid arthritis) can cause drug-induced myasthenia. If the drug is discontinued, the myasthenia-like syndrome resolves. Although TIA and stroke must be considered in the diagnosis, it is very unusual for ischemia to produce diplopia alone. Often, other neurological symptoms are present. Graves ophthalmopathy must always be considered when a patient has diplopia. Often, physical signs of Graves disease, such as the Graves stare, will suggest a diagnosis of thyroid disease.

The first diagnostic test is the Tensilon test. When clinical signs are present (not just subjective diplopia), the Tensilon test can confirm the clinical diagnosis. Tensilon (edrophonium) is a short-acting acetylcholinesterase inhibitor that acts to prolong the effects of acetylcholine at the postsynaptic neuromuscular junction. This will reverse the weakness transiently. A positive test, then, would be improvement in clinical signs. A second test is the acetylcholine receptor antibody test. It is positive in 50% of patients with ocular myasthenia, and positive in 90% of patients with generalized myasthenia. In this case (ocular symptoms only), it would be a second-line test. However, the only manufacturer of edrophonium (Tensilon) stopped producing it in February 2008. So once supplies are exhausted, only the antibody test is available. CT of the chest would be indicated to eliminate the possibility of a thymoma, which is present in about 15% of patients with myasthenia gravis. EMG may be performed as a confirmatory test as well. The classic EMG finding in myasthenia gravis is the electro-decremental response to repetitive stimulation. An MRI of the brain would not be needed.

Board Testing Point: Recognize the clinical features of myasthenia gravis and know how to diagnose the disease.

439. Answer: C

Answer: Oxygen.
Intranasal oxygen therapy is the most effective abortive remedy. Delivered for about 15–20 mins. If oxygen is not available, triptans can be used to abort the headache. Verapramil, prednisone, topiramate, and lithium can be used for **prophylactic** treatment.

Board Testing Point: Know appropriate abortive therapies for cluster headache.

RHEUMATOLOGY

440. Answer: D

Answer: Joint hypermobility syndrome.
This patient fulfills Beighton and Brighton criteria for joint hypermobility syndrome—the Beighton score is based on:

- Being able to bend the thumb to the forearm (1 point each per thumb)
- Hyperextension of the fingers (1 point each for right and left hand)
- Hyperextension of the elbows (1 point each per elbow)
- Hyperextension of the knees (1 point each per knee)
- Being able to touch the palms to the floor while standing with knees extended (1 point)

A score of 4/9 or higher suggests hypermobility.

This patient's history and exam do not suggest an inflammatory process, thus excluding rheumatoid arthritis and seronegative spondyloarthritis. She also does not fulfill criteria for fibromyalgia. While she may develop secondary osteoarthritis due to joint hypermobility, this is not the best answer for the case scenario.

Board Testing Point: Recognize joint hypermobility syndrome as a common cause of arthralgia.

441. Answer: C

Answer: Trimethoprim/sulfamethoxazole (TMP/SMX).
Avoid prescribing trimethoprim/sulfamethoxazole (TMP/SMX) in patients on methotrexate due to risk for methotrexate toxicity. TMX/SMX can reduce renal clearance of methotrexate as well as contribute to heighten anti-folate effects. Penicillins can also reduce the clearance of methotrexate, and patients should be closely monitored while on the antibiotic. While the other antibiotics listed can interact with methotrexate to some degree, they can and have been used safely with methotrexate.

Board Testing Point: Know potential drug interactions with common medications and anti-rheumatic drugs.

442. Answer: D

Answer: Get an HLA-B*5801 gene marker.
The 2012 ACR gout management guidelines indicate that prior to initiating allopurinol, consider HLA-B*5801 screening in selected patients, specifically those higher-risk sub-populations for severe allopurinol hypersensitivity reaction (e.g., Koreans with stage 3 or worse CKD; Han Chinese and Thai irrespective of renal function). The guidelines also note that initial allopurinol dose should not exceed 100 mg/day (and for those with CKD stage 4 or worse, no higher than 50 mg/day); allopurinol dose should be titrated every 2–5 weeks to achieve target uric acid goal < 6.0 mg/dL. HLA-B*51 gene marker is thought to predispose patients to Behçet syndrome. HLA-B*27 gene marker predisposes patients to spondyloarthropathies.

Board Testing Point: Understand that certain populations are at higher risk for allopurinol hypersensitivity.

443. Answer: A

Answer: Classic polyarteritis nodosa (PAN).
Visceral angiography may be necessary to establish this diagnosis. Biopsy of skin, kidney, or other tissues should demonstrate the typical fibrinoid necrosis. Although often suggested otherwise in various sources, the association of the ANCA antibodies is not with this entity but with the following:

p-ANCA

1) Microscopic polyarteritis (MPA): involvement of venules, capillaries, arterioles
2) Churg-Strauss: eosinophilia

c-ANCA

1) Granulomatosis with polyangiitis (Wegener's): upper respiratory involvement (sinuses)

Classic PAN affecting medium-sized arteries is usually not associated with ANCA markers at all. If an antibody association is present, there may be evidence for hepatitis response in some patients.

Board Testing Point: Recognize the clinical findings of polyarteritis nodosa.

444. Answer: D

Answer: Adult-onset Still's disease.
Adult-onset Still's disease (AOSD) is a common cause of fever of unknown origin. It is characterized by quotidian fever (daily spikes in temperature), arthritis (typically symmetric), and an evanescent rash that is a maculopapular rash, often salmon colored and typically occurs with the fever. Serositis, sore throat, myalgias are also common manifestions of AOSD. Laboratory abnormalities include: elevated ferritin, white blood cell count, ESR, and abnormal liver function tests.

The other diagnoses are unlikely. Whipple disease generally occurs in middle-age/elderly males and is caused by infection with *Tropheryma whipplei*; diarrhea with large joint involvement is a predominant symptom of Whipple diasease. While the ANA is low-positive, this patient's symptoms are not consistent with SLE. Reactive arthritis, which is manifested by arthritis, conjunctivitis, and urethritis, preceded by infection, is incorrect. You would expect a history of sexually-transmitted disease or penile discharge for gonococcal arthritis.

Board Testing Point: Recognize the clinical features of adult-onset Still's disease.

445. Answer: A

Answer: Sjögren syndrome with non-Hodgkin lymphoma.
With the sicca symptoms, +ANA, +SSA, the patient obviously has Sjögren syndrome. The lymph nodes sound ominous in the description, and there is a significantly increased risk of non-Hodgkin lymphoma in patients with Sjögren syndrome; this is the best answer for the question. In general, there is a higher risk of non-Hodgkin lymphoma with most of the connective tissue disease processes.

Board Testing Point: Recognize that Sjögren's patients have a higher risk of non-Hodgkin lymphoma.

446. Answer: C

Answer: Anti-histone antibody.
Anti-SCL70 is found in 8% of scleroderma patients with diffuse progressive disease. ANAs are frequently found in patients with scleroderma. Anti-centromere antibody is often found with CREST syndrome, which is limited cutaneous disease. Rheumatoid factors are nonspecific in this situation, but anti-histone antibodies are usually found in drug-induced lupus.

Board Testing Point: Recognize that scleroderma is associated with finding a positive ANA, anti-SCL70, anti-centromere antibody, and RF.

447. Answer: E

Answer: Prednisone 15 mg/day.
Her symptoms are typical of polymyalgia rheumatica: limb-girdle myalgia but no muscle weakness on physical exam, anemia, and elevated ESR. Low doses of prednisone (10 mg to 20 mg/day) are used for PMR alone while high doses of 60 mg/day of prednisone is for PMR with evidence of giant cell arteritis. Gabapentin would be used for her peripheral neuropathy. TCAs are used for nonarticular rheumatism such as fibromyalgia, which would not have an elevated ESR.

Board Testing Point: Recognize the clinical features of polymyalgia rheumatica and the appropriate dose of prednisone for treatment.

448. Answer: B

Answer: Physical therapy.
The patient has several risk factors for frozen shoulder syndrome, and the appropriate treatment is aggressive physical therapy. Perhaps non-steroidals could be used, but physical therapy is the first option. A steroid injection would not help this adhesive capsulitis. Prednisone is not indicated and would worsen this patient's diabetes.

Board Testing Point: Recognize frozen shoulder (adhesive capsulitis) and that physical therapy is the best treatment.

449. Answer: C

Answer: CT scan of SI joints.
The patient has a seronegative spondyloarthropathy (probable ankylosing spondylitis) and is likely to be HLA-B27-positive, but this is very nonspecific and not diagnostic. CT scan of the SI joints is very useful for showing bony erosive changes at the sacroiliac joints. An MRI of the lumbar spine and chest x-ray would be indicated for late changes of AS on physical exam.

Board Testing Point: Recognize the clinical features of spondyloarthropathy and the need to determine erosive sacroiliitis.

450. Answer: A

Answer: Vitamin B_6.
The inappropriate choice is vitamin B_6. The patient seems to have clinical evidence suggestive of carpal tunnel entrapment. Release, splint, and corticosteroid injection are all appropriate. Vitamin B_6 has been studied and has been shown not to be effective.

Board Testing Point: Recognize carpal tunnel entrapment and its appropriate therapies.

451. Answer: B

Answer: Rapidly progressive glomerulonephritis with crescents.
This patient clearly has granulomatosis with polyangiitis (Wegener's) with the characteristic c-ANCA titer. With the proliferative sediment, trace proteinuria, and the rapid increase in creatinine, RPGN is the likely diagnosis. Minimal change usually is milder. Membranous nephropathy is associated with massive proteinuria (nephrotic syndrome). Focal sclerosis is usually seen in HIV and IV drug abusers.

Board Testing Point: Recognize that granulomatosis with polyangiitis (Wegener's) is likely to lead to rapidly progressive glomerulonephritis.

452. Answer: E

Answer: Sputum for AFB.
The anti-TNF drugs (infliximab) have been associated with a higher risk of tuberculosis. All patients beginning biologic therapy, especially anti-TNF drugs, must have a chest x-ray and PPD done prior to the commencement of these drugs. The other tests would not identify *Mycobacterium tuberculosis*.

Board Testing Point: Recognize that infliximab use is associated with an increased risk of tuberculosis.

453. Answer: A

Answer: Positive anti-centromere antibodies.
She has had stable Raynaud's for 10 years. Therefore, to suddenly now develop a connective tissue disease process is unlikely. The dilated capillaries are of concern, but not present in all of her digits. ANA's are found in 20% of patients with primary Raynaud's. Anti-centromere is seen in CREST. Rheumatoid factor is 85% specific for rheumatoid arthritis, but it can also be false-positive for other conditions. ESR would be normal with primary Raynaud disease.

Board Testing Point: Recognize the clinical features and labs associated with Raynaud disease.

454. Answer: C

Answer: Occasional ECHO to estimate pulmonary pressure.
This patient has CREST syndrome, a limited cutaneous form of scleroderma. While the prognosis is generally regarded as one of the more benign variants of scleroderma, nevertheless, pulmonary HTN is well described. Therefore, it would be important to look for the early presence of pulmonary HTN, particularly given the newer groups of medications that could potentially arrest this. A small bowel follow-through would be indicated for signs of pseudo-obstruction of the small bowel, which this patient does not have. ANA titers do not correlate with disease activity. An SPEP is not indicated for scleroderma patients.

Board Testing Point: Recognize the need to follow patients with CREST syndrome for development of pulmonary hypertension.

455. Answer: A

Answer: IV immunoglobulin.
The "incorrect" therapy would be IV immunoglobulin. IVIG is indicated for refractory cases of dermatomyositis, not as initial therapy. This patient obviously has dermatomyositis and will require long-term corticosteroid therapy. According to the latest recommendations of the American College of Rheumatology, any patient requiring prednisone at a dose of 5 mg qd or greater for a period of 3 months or longer will require a bisphosphonate. Bone loss is dramatic in the first few weeks after initiating glucocorticoids, particularly at higher doses. However, dramatic bone loss occurs even at a relatively low dose of 7.5 mg qd. Calcium is also used as adjunctive therapy with bisphosphonates.

Board Testing Point: Know that agents to prevent bone loss are indicated in patients requiring long-term corticosteroid use.

456. Answer: C

Answer: Diabetic-limited joint mobility syndrome.
This patient has classic features of diabetic-limited joint mobility syndrome to include a positive prayer's sign, history of presumed "frozen shoulder syndrome," Dupuytren contractures, and carpal tunnel syndrome. She has pseudoscleroderma of Buschke. Other features include rotator cuff tendinitis, rotator cuff calcification, and bicipital tendinitis. If the stenosing tenosynovitis is caught early, which is responsible for her triggering, then a local corticosteroid injection is highly appropriate. Of course, there may be a temporary loss of diabetic control. However, if the stenosis of her tendon sheaths is fairly chronic, then a simple operative procedure by a hand surgeon would be appropriate.

Board Testing Point: Be able to discern diabetic-limited joint mobility syndrome in an appropriate patient scenario.

457. Answer: D

Answer: Repeat ANA, anti-dsDNA titers, anti-centromere, and anti-SCL70.
The patient most likely has primary Raynaud disease. Approximately 20% of younger women with primary Raynaud's have a positive ANA, and this is not always an appropriate screening test. However, given the fact that her ANA is known to be positive, it would be appropriate and reassuring to exclude a secondary process. Her symptoms do not particularly suggest a connective tissue disease process, but a repeat ANA would be appropriate because of variations from lab to lab. The specific serologies for lupus, including anti-dsDNA and SM, would be reasonable. So, too, would be an anti-centromere to rule out CREST and an anti-SCL70 to exclude diffuse systemic sclerosis. If these last 2 tests were found to be positive, then a further screening to include manometry, ECHO, etc., would be appropriate. The negative vital capillaroscopy and normal Allen's test (positive blood flow) is indeed reassuring.

Board Testing Point: Recognize that you must exclude other etiologies before making the diagnosis of primary Raynaud disease.

458. Answer: C

Answer: Check baseline labs to include CBC, sed rate, RF, and aspirate one of the knees.
This patient has a classic reactive arthritis, probably acquired through a GI route. She provides no history to suggest any other reactive features to include urethritis or conjunctivitis. IV antibiotics would obviously have been inappropriate. It would be more appropriate to aspirate the joint and have baseline labs checked before proceeding to systemic corticosteroids or local joint injection.

Board Testing Point: Recognize the clinical features of a reactive arthritis and the basic laboratory workup to rule out other more serious etiologies.

459. Answer: D

Answer: Prednisone 10 mg qd.
This patient has osteoarthritis, which can be progressive in some patients. The "incorrect" therapeutic option would be prednisone 10 mg qd. This patient is elderly and has had a previous history of peptic ulcer and, therefore, is classically at risk for life-threatening GI bleed. The COX-2 inhibitors have been developed specifically for this purpose, and there are outcome studies to demonstrate a significant reduction in life-threatening GI bleeds with this class of drugs. However, their cardiovascular effects have resulted in many being removed from the market with only celecoxib remaining. Because of this, many recommend NSAIDs with proton pump inhibitors instead, although NSAIDs have recently been shown to increase cardiovascular risk as well with the exception of naprosyn. Hydrocodone is obviously addictive and is the last option for this patient. There is no reason to give him systemic corticosteroid therapy.

Board Testing Point: Recognize that oral corticosteroid has no use in the treatment of osteoarthritis.

460. Answer: B

Answer: CT scan of the SI joints.
The patient has a seronegative spondyloarthropathy probably due to inflammatory bowel disease (enteropathic spondyloarthropathy). CT scan would be inappropriate. This patient has classic symptoms of inflammatory back pain, suggesting a spondyloarthropahty. An MRI of the SI joints has become the study of choice in the last decade. While early changes may be missed on a simple film of the LS-spine and SI joints and a CT scan is highly sensitive for erosive changes in the SI joints, most do not recommend CT scan because of the increased gonadal radiation associated with this modality. MRI of the lumbosacral spine would also pick up a bamboo spine correlating with his abnormal Schober's test. Sub-clinical uveitis needs to be excluded in this patient. His GI symptoms certainly suggest that he has inflammatory bowel disease, which definitely could be related to his musculoskeletal symptoms. Thus, the need for colonoscopy.

Board Testing Point: Recognize the clinical features of seronegative spondyloarthropathy (enteropathic spondyloarthropathy) and know what tests are needed/recommended for evaluation.

461. Answer: B

Answer: Bisphosphonate.
She has polymyalgia rheumatica (PMR). Any patient who is going to be on prednisone at a dose of $>$ 5 mg qd for longer than 3 months should be placed on a bisphosphonate as prophylaxis against glucocorticoid-induced osteoporosis (GIOP) with potential for fractures.These are current American College of Rheumatology recommendations for GIOP. For most PMR patients, the average patient requires glucocorticoid therapy for about 1 year. SERMs and calcitonin have not clinically been demonstrated to prevent glucocorticoid-induced osteoporosis. Estrogen would help but is no longer recommended because of the increased risk of breast cancer and stroke.

Board Testing Point: Recognize that patients on long-term glucocorticoid therapy are at increased risk for developing osteoporosis and resultant fractures.

462. Answer: B

Answer: Ferritin and calcium levels.
The history of intermittent inflammatory arthritis and evidence of chondrocalcinosis suggest a diagnosis of calcium pyrophosphate deposition disease (CPPD). In the presence of hooked or bulky osteophytes in the 2nd and 3rd MCP joints, hemochromatosis should be considered. During an acute flare, synovial fluid may reveal CPPD crystals, which are positively birefringent. Hemochromatosis and hyperparathyroidism are 2 diseases strongly associated with CPPD. A CT scan of the SI joint would not be helpful because suspicion of a seronegative spondyloarthritis is low. A bone scan may show inflamed joints but would not be specific to help aid in diagnosis. Anti-Jo-1 occurs in the setting of myositis and would not be helpful in this case.

Board Testing Point: Recognize the clinical features of calcium pyrophosphate deposition disease, and understand the need to screen for hemochromatosis and hyperparathyroidism.

463. Answer: D

Answer: Dermatomyositis.
His exam is consistent with dermatomyositis. Note that he has Gottron papules on his knuckles, which is the most specific finding for this disease. The elevated aldolase is helpful; so too is the proximal muscle weakness. Another classic finding (but which he doesn't have) is the "heliotrope" rash on the upper eyelids. Remember the ANA is nonspecific and can be seen in other autoimmune diseases as well as in healthy individuals. The patient does not fulfill criteria for scleroderma, rheumatoid arthritis, or SLE. Given the abnormal labs and exam, he has more than just chronic fatigue syndrome.

Board Testing Point: Recognize the clinical features of dermatomyositis.

464. Answer: C

Answer: Impingement syndrome.
This refers to compression of the subacromial bursa or regional tendons in the space between the acromion and the humeral head. The biceps tendon and all the rotator cuff tendons go through this area. The passive abduction to 90 degrees causing pain in the deltoid region is the test that nails this one. A rotator cuff tear would cause more pain during active abduction than passive abduction. Bursitis of the subacromial bursa would do the same thing. Osteoarthritis of the shoulder is very rare. A thoracic outlet syndrome would cause pain that extends from the base of the neck, over the top of the shoulder, and down the arm.

Board Testing Point: Recognize the clinical manifestations of impingement syndrome.

465. Answer: A

Answer: *Mycobacterium marinum.*
Note that he has a chronic process x 2 years. He sustained an injury in water. Put the two together and you come up with *Mycobacterium marinum*! Note, it is common for you **not** to be able to culture this organism. Again, the water exposure is the kicker here. Think of the other organisms if the environmental exposure is right: *Nocardia*—soil; *Blastomyces*—soil or lumber; *Sporothrix*—gardens or plants.

Board Testing Point: Recognize the clinical features of *Mycobacterium marinum*.

466. Answer: E

Answer: Hepatitis C serology.
This patient has cryoglobulinemia. It is mixed due to the abnormally high rheumatoid factor binding to either monoclonal or polyclonal IgG. Vasculitis with purpura is the most common presentation for mixed cryoglobulinemia. Hepatitis C has a very strong association with mixed cryoglobulinemia! In one study, 86% of cryoglobulinemics were positive for hepatitis C! The monoclonal type is due to multiple myeloma or Waldenström macroglobulinemia—with this you would expect to see severe hemolytic anemia and something in the history like Raynaud's or cyanosis with exposure to cold.

Board Testing Point: Recognize the association between hepatitis C and cryoglobulinemia.

467. Answer: B

Answer: Avascular necrosis of the hip.
Up to 1/3 of SLE patients on chronic steroids will develop avascular necrosis of a hip. Best way to diagnose it is with an MRI. The acute onset makes you steer away from the osteomyelitis diagnose. A fracture should have been seen on plain film.

Board Testing Point: Recognize that avascular necrosis of the hip is more likely to occur in patients who have been on chronic steroids.

468. Answer: B

Answer: Dual-energy x-ray absorptiometry.
Commonly known as DXA, this is the quickest method. Precision of the DXA approaches 1–2%. The quantitative CT scan and dual photon absorptiometry take a lot of time. The CT scan has the drawback of giving a lot of radiation.

Board Testing Point: Know that DXA scan is the test of choice for screening for osteoporosis.

469. Answer: D

Answer: Loss of lower esophageal sphincter function.
Note that loss of lower espohageal sphincter function is the most common abnormality seen in patients with systemic sclerosis. The rest of the abnormalities listed are uncommon in this condition.

Board Testing Point: Recognize that loss of lower esophageal sphincter function is a common finding on barium swallow in a patient with systemic sclerosis.

470. Answer: C

Answer: Behçet syndrome examination shows significant arthritis of his bilateral knees.
Behçet syndrome is a recurrent disease of unknown etiology and is characterized by painful oral and genital ulcers, eye inflammation, arthritis; CNS symptoms (aseptic meningitis) with fever, abdominal complaints and thombophlebitis also can be seen in this disease. These symptoms can mimic inflammatory bowel disease (IBD). While peripheral neuropathies are common with IBD, CNS involvement is not. Whipple disease is associated with arthritis, abdominal pain, and CNS disease, but typically seen in older males. A negative ANA virtually excludes the diagnosis of SLE.

Board Testing Point: Recognize the clinical features of Behçet syndrome.

471. Answer: C

Answer: Allopurinol.
You would **not** use allopurinol for treatment of acute gouty arthritis! The nonsteroidal antiinflammatory drugs, oral colchicine (IV is no longer available in the U.S.), or oral or intraarticular steroids can be used in the acute presentation. Colchicine inhibits neutrophil activation by inhibiting crystal-induced protein tyrosine phosphorylation. Many patients, because of the GI side effects, do not tolerate oral colchicine. Allopurinol, remember, is for long-term management of gout; because it can **prolong** an attack, it should not be started for acute gout.

Board Testing Point: Recognize different treatment options for acute gout.

472. Answer: E

Answer: Pseudogout.
Calcium pyrophosphate dihydrate (CPPD) crystals cause chondrocalcinosis (calcium in the cartilage). Pseudogout is the term used for the acute presentation of the disease. The crystals of pseudogout have weakly positive birefringence on compensated polarized light microscopy as opposed to gout where the crystals have strongly negative birefringence under polarized light.

Board Testing Point: Recognize the clinical features of pseudogout.

473. Answer: A

Answer: Reactive arthritis.
Reactive arthritis (formerly Reiter syndrome) classically presents with a triad of urethritis, conjunctivitis, and arthritis and is the best answer for this question. The arthritis usually involves the large joint of the lower extremities and is asymmetrical. Causes of reactive arthritis are genitourinary infections from *Chlamydia* or *Ureaplasma* and gastrointestinal infections due to *Salmonella*, *Shigella*, *Yersinia*, *Klebsiella*, and *Campylobacter*.

Board Testing Point: Recognize the clinical features of reactive arthritis.

474. Answer: D

Answer: Raynaud phenomenon.
Raynaud phenomenon is **not** used as a criterion to classify systemic lupus erythematosus. **Be sure** you know the ACR classification criteria for SLE. On the exam, they will give you a patient with nonspecific findings, and you will have to know to find 4 or more of the 11 that are SLE-specific. The 11 are: photosensitivity, blood changes (anemia, leukopenia, etc.), renal disease, +ANA, +anti-dsDNA or anti-Sm antibody or antiphospholipid antibody, arthritis, malar rash, discoid rash, neuropsychiatric features (psychosis, seizures), oral lesions, and serositis.

Board Testing Point: Know the ACR classification criteria for SLE.

475. Answer: B

Answer: Heberden node.
Heberden and Bouchard nodes are **not** seen in rheumatoid arthritis but are seen in **osteoarthritis**. Heberden nodes are enlargement of the DIP joint, and Bouchard nodes are bony enlargement of the PIP joints. All of the other findings listed are consistent with long-standing rheumatoid arthritis.

Board Testing Point: Recognize the clinical features that distinguish rheumatoid arthritis from osteoarthritis.

476. Answer: A

Answer: dsDNA antibody.
This patient likely has systemic lupus erythematosus. As active as her disease is, it would be good to check and see if she is dsDNA antibody-positive, which test is highly associated with lupus nephritis. The presence of a dsDNA would confirm the diagnosis of SLE in this patient. The anti-Sm antibody is specific for SLE. The RNP antibody is mainly seen with mixed connective tissue disease but can be found in SLE on occasion. The SSA (Ro) antibody is more helpful with neonatal lupus, Sjögren syndrome, and systemic sclerosis. Anti-histone is used to differentiate drug-induced lupus (but can be seen also in SLE). c-ANCA is seen with granulomatosis with polyangiitis (Wegener's).

Board Testing Point: Recognize clinical features of SLE, and know that anti-dsDNA antibody is associated with renal disease.

477. Answer: E

Answer: X-rays of the sacroiliac joints are indicated.
This man likely has ankylosing spondylitis based on his history and physical examination. The x-ray findings in patients with ankylosing spondylitis can include sacroiliitis, calcification of the longitudinal ligaments and syndesmophytes.

Note: It would be rare to find an ankylosing spondylitis patient who has spondylitis without sacroiliitis! The diagnosis must be differentiated from inflammatory bowel disease or psoriasis, which can give you similar findings as far as the arthropathy and sacroiliitis.

Board Testing Point: Recognize the clinical features of ankylosing spondylitis.

478. Answer: C

Answer: Gout.
His x-ray findings are consistent with long-standing gout. Remember, the 1st metatarsophalangeal joint is the most common joint to be involved. Also, he has chronic tophaceous gout with the findings of the tophaceous deposits of monosodium urate (negatively birefringent crystals!) at his olecranon bursae. The other sites for these are the Achilles tendons and the external ear. Tophi are painless, but their presence in and around joints can limit joint mobility.

Board Testing Point: Recognize the clinical features of gout.

479. Answer: B

Answer: Tell her that her risk of osteoporosis is very low, and no testing is required at this time.
This patient is at low risk for fracture, and no further testing is required. Current guidelines for bone density screening indicate that the following individuals be tested:

a) Women age 65 and older and men age 70 and older, regardless of clinical risk factors
b) Younger postmenopausal women and men age 50–69 about whom you have concern based on their clinical risk factor profile
c) Women in the menopausal transition if there is a specific risk factor associated with increased fracture risk such as low body weight, prior low-trauma fracture, or high-risk medication
d) Adults who have a fracture after age 50, adults with a condition (e.g., rheumatoid arthritis) or taking a medication (e.g., glucocorticoids in a daily dose ≥ 5 mg prednisone or equivalent for ≥ 3 months) associated with low bone mass or bone loss
e) Anyone being considered for pharmacologic therapy for osteoporosis
f) Anyone being treated for osteoporosis—to monitor treatment effect
g) Anyone not receiving therapy in whom evidence of bone loss would lead to treatment

Board Testing Point: Recognize who should be screened for osteoporosis.

480. Answer: A

Answer: Chronic oral steroid use.
With his asthma history, you have to wonder if he is on chronic steroids. These will induce early osteoporosis, especially in men. The other drugs listed are not associated with early osteoporosis. Other risk factors for his osteoporosis can include hypogonadism.

Board Testing Point: Recognize the association of chronic oral steroid use with osteoporosis.

481. Answer: B

Answer: Corticosteroid phonopheresis into the carpal tunnel.
Therapeutic ultrasound using phonopheresis with steroids or NSAIDs have been found to be effective in managing patients with carpal tunnel syndrome. The other choices are not indicated. Repeating the EMG/NCS would not help at this point.

Board Testing Point: Recognize that conservative measures to managing carpal tunnel syndrome include: splints, injectable/oral steroids, NSAIDs, and phonopheresis with therapeutic ultrasound.

482. Answer: B

Answer: Exertional chest pain relieved with rest.
Obviously, this woman is having pain, which must make you think about angina or coronary disease syndromes. All of the other findings are seen with osteoporosis. The pulmonary dysfunction can occur as the total lung capacity is reduced by changes in the architecture of the thorax due to disease progression and worsening dorsal kyphosis and cervical lordosis.

Board Testing Point: Recognize that exertional chest pain is not associated with osteoporosis.

483. Answer: D

Answer: Cyclosporine.
This patient has typical clinical features of gout: acute onset of severe foot pain. He is on cyclosporine, a drug that increases uric acid levels and frequently can cause gout. Although aspirin in low doses can slightly increase gout risk, cyclosporine is much more likely (up to 30% develop gout). Alcohol can also increase the risk of gout, but no history of alcohol use is given in this case.

Board Testing Point: Recognize the clinical features of gout and that cyclosporine may induce an acute attack.

484. Answer: E

Answer: Adverse effect due to ciprofloxacin.
This patient develops Achilles tendon pain after a ski vacation. An acute injury from skiing is a possibility, but in the setting of prolonged ciprofloxacin use, quinolone-induced tendonitis/tendon injury is more likely. Tendon rupture related to quinolone use has been well documented in the literature, with the most cases attributed to ciprofloxacin. It is a side effect of the drug class and not related to any drug interactions.

Board Testing Point: Recognize the association of Achilles tendon rupture with use of quinolones.

485. Answer: C

Answer: Rheumatoid arthritis.
This patient has tophaceous gout; notice the white crystals on a distended olecranon bursa. Gout has been associated with risks for renal insufficiency, cardiovascular morbidity/mortality, metabolic syndrome, and disability. There has not been an association of gout with rheumatoid arthritis—it is generally believed that patients who have rheumatoid arthritis have a lower risk for gout and vice versa—though both conditions have been reported in the same patient before.

Board Testing Point: Know the associated co-morbidities that can be seen with gout.

486. Answer: B

Answer: Start allopurinol and titrate to serum uric acid < 6.0 mg/dL.
Per the American College of Rheumatology 2012 gout management guidelines, all patients with gout should be counseled about dietary and lifestyle changes, but this is difficult for most patients to accomplish. However, urate lowering therapy (ULT) is most effective in the management of gout and should be initiated in those who have 2 or more gout attacks, with goal uric acid < 6.0 mg/dL in patients without tophi; for those with tophi, setting the goal uric acid < 5.0 mg/dL will accelerate the dissolution of tophi. Antiinflammatory prophylaxis with **low**-dose NSAIDs or **oral** colchicine is indicated when initiating urate lowering therapy. Duration of prophylaxis should be 6 months or 3 months after goal uric acid is achieved if there is no history of tophi. There is no history of nephrolithiasis in this patient for alkalinization of urine.

Board Testing Point: Understand urate lowering therapy (ULT) as most effective in the management of gout.

487. Answer: D

Answer: HLA-B27.
Suspicion for a seronegative spondyloarthritis is low, and ordering an HLA-B27 would not be indicated in evaluating this patient's pain. Recognize that HLA-B27 is not diagnostic for ankylosing spondylitis since it is also found in 8% of normal healthy Caucasians. Note the patient's pain is consistent with mechanical pain (morning stiffness < 30 min, worse with activity, improves with rest, and worse in late afternoon/evenings) rather than inflammatory pain (mornings are worse, morning stiffness lasts > 45 min, pain improves with activity). A testosterone level would be useful for this patient—note that he has been on long-term narcotics, which can lower testosterone levels. Hypogonadism can mimic fibromyalgia in male patients. Thyroid function tests, sleep study, and back x-rays would be useful tests and indicated in evaluating this patient.

Board Testing Point: Be able to distinguish inflammatory from mechanical back pain.

488. Answer: B

Answer: Rheumatoid arthritis (RA).
The photo shows evidence of an inflammatory arthritis (look at the patient's right 3rd digit and left 4th digit). This patient likely has seronegative rheumatoid arthritis. Seronegativity occurs in about 20% of patients who have rheumatoid arthritis.

While patients with SLE may present with an inflammatory arthritis, the ANA is negative in this patient, and she does not have other signs/symptoms of SLE. Gout is an incorrect answer because it is highly unlikely for gout to occur in a menstruating female. Hand OA is also incorrect because typically this disease affects the distal interphalangeal joints (DIPs) in older patients.

Board Testing Point: Recognize manifestations of rheumatoid arthritis.

489. Answer: A

Answer: Methotrexate pneumonitis.
Methotrexate pneumonitis is a rare drug hypersensitivity that typically occurs within the first year of use. Beacause this patient had been stable on his current medication regimen for at least 7 years, methotrexate pneumonitis is unlikely to be the reason for his shortness of breath. Rheumatoid lung or interstitial lung disease can be seen with longstanding RA and can contribute to symptoms of shortness of breath along with infection and heart disease. Maintain vigilance for typical and atypical infections in patients who are immunosuppressed. Rheumatoid arthritis is a recognized risk factor for coronary artery disease and congestive heart failure; keep this in mind when considering the differential diagnosis of dyspnea in a patient with rheumatoid arthritis.

Board Testing Point: Understand that methotrexate pneumonitis is rare and that other etiologies of dyspnea in a patient with rheumatoid arthritis should be considered.

490. Answer: A

Answer: Giant cell arteritis.
Giant cell arteritis (GCA) can present with diplopia, scalp tenderness, headaches, jaw claudication, weight loss, low-grade fever, amaurosis fugax, and polymyalgia rheumatic symptoms of the shoulder/hip regions. Note that GCA is a large vessel vasculitis and often an elevated ESR and normochromic, normocytic anemia is evident. While patients and their spouses like to offer their opinion on what they think their symptoms are due to, keep in mind the patterns of certain diseases. While the other choices are remote differential possibilities, GCA is the best answer based on history, exam and labs.

Board Testing Point: Recognize the common manifestations of GCA.

491. Answer: B

Answer: Hydroxychloroquine.
The treatment of RA in pregnancy can be difficult. Most medications must be discontinued months prior to conception in order to minimize the risk of affecting fetal development. Methotrexate is among the most well known to be contraindicated with pregnancy, classified as category X for a syndrome consisting of skeletal, CNS, and cardiac abnormalities. NSAIDs should be avoided because this can interfere with implantation of the embryo. Prednisone use would increase the risk of the development of cleft palate, though sometimes it can be used depending on the clinical scenario. Biologic DMARDs are not well studied in terms of fetal risk and are not recommended in pregnancy, even though risk has not been clearly demonstrated. Hydroxychloroquine has not been demonstrated to have any fetal effects. Women with RA can be enrolled in a registry to monitor for fetal effects while on hydroxychloroquine during their pregnancy.

Board Testing Point: Recognize treatments for rheumatoid arthritis that are safe to continue in pregnancy.

492. Answer: B

Answer: Allopurinol.
This is the classic presentation for gout. The **negatively** birefringent crystals in the joint fluid confirm the diagnosis.

Allopurinol and azathioprine together is potentially a dangerous combination. Allopurinol can interfere with the metabolism of azathioprine, increasing the risk for bone marrow toxicity. If the combination cannot be avoided, the dose of azathioprine should be reduced by 25% of the recommended dose and the patient's blood count be carefully monitored.

Remember that allopurinol is not started as treatment for acute gout. It is a longer-term urate-lowering agent like febuxostat, probenecid, and pegloticase. Allopurinol and fuboxostat are xanthine oxidase inhibitors and a similar drug interaction can be seen with azathioprine and febuxostat.

So, for an autoimmune patient on azathioprine who presents with gout, either avoid xanthine oxidase inhibitors or switch their azathioprine to another agent.

The other medications listed above are safe to use in this patient but know that prednisone and acetaminophen are inappropriate for prophylaxis of gout.

Board Testing Point: Know common drug interactions and dose adjustments for azathioprine when indicated.

ALLERGY / IMMUNOLOGY

493. Answer: B

Answer: Surface immunoglobulin M.
Remember that surface immunoglobulin M is the first immunoglobulin class produced. IgM is the default immunoglobulin. The other immunoglobulin isotypes are produced after B-cell class switching.

Board Testing Point: Remember that surface immunoglobulin M is the first immunoglobulin class produced during B-cell development.

494. Answer: A

Answer: C1 esterase inhibitor.
The patient most likely has hereditary angioedema (HAE). Bradykinin is the mediator responsible for angioedema in patients with HAE. Reduced levels or low functional levels of C1 esterase inhibitor leads to excessive bradykinin release and angioedema. C1 esterase inhibitor replacement protein (C1INHRP) was approved in October 2008 for treatment of acute attacks of HAE.

C5A is incorrect because it is an anaphylatoxin that can induce angioedema episodes. Low C5A levels would not be associated with angioedema. IgE is a nonspecifc marker of allergic disease. Low surface immunoglobulin A would not be associated with angioedema. Bradykinin is not correct because quite the contrary, high (not low) levels of bradykinin are present in plasma of patients with HAE.

Board Testing Point: Recognize the clinical features of C1 esterase inhibitor deficiency (hereditary angioedema).

495. Answer: A

Answer: Ataxia-telangiectasia.
Ataxia-telangiectasia (AT) is a rare autosomal recessive disorder characterized by neurodegeneration, immunodeficiency, extreme sensitivity to radiation and predisposition to cancer. The progressive cerebellar ataxia and telangiectasias are hallmarks of this disease. The gene responsible (ATM) is located on chromosome 11. The defect in the ATM gene results in an inability to repair damaged DNA. Patients with AT have defects in both humoral and cellular immunity, and develop recurrent sinopulmonary infections and chronic lung disease (bronchiectasis). Aspiration pneumonia occurs as a result of defects in chewing and swallowing due to progressive neurological impairment.

Severe combined immunodeficiency (SCID) is incorrect because SCID is not associated with progressive cerebellar ataxia. An abnormality on chromosome 12 is incorrect because the gene for AT is located on the long arm of chromosome 11 (not 12). Friedreich ataxia is an autosomal recessive disorder characterized by progressive limb and gait ataxia, sensory loss, weakness, and dysarthria. Unlike ataxia-telangiectasia, there are no associated defects in immune function. Cystic fibrosis (CF) is an autosomal recessive disorder characterized by mutations in the CF transmembrane conductance regulator (CFTR) gene, which results in abnormal transport of sodium and chloride across an epithelium. Mucosal obstruction of the exocrine glands results in lung, liver, pancreatic, and intestinal disease. CF is not associated with neurodeneration and progressive ataxia.

Board Testing Point: Recognize the clinical features of ataxia-telangiectasia.

496. Answer: B

Answer: Direct activation of mediator release from mast cells, basophils, or both.
The patient is having anaphylaxis to radiocontrast media. Anaphylaxis typically occurs through an IgE-mediated mechanism, most commonly triggered by bee stings, foods, and latex. Radiocontrast media, however, can trigger anaphylaxis through an IgE-independent mechanism, directly activating mast cells and basophils to release the mediators of anaphylaxis. Traditionally, this type of reaction has been referred to as **anaphylactoid** reactions. Anaphylaxis due to penicillin and other antibiotics is due to IgE recognition of protein-hapten conjugants. Finally, dialysis can induce anaphylaxis with complement activation.

Board Testing Point: Recognize the clinical features and mechanism for anaphylaxis of radiocontrast dye.

497. Answer: B

Answer: Systemic mastocytosis.
She has a syndrome characterized by mast cell infiltration of the skin (the small bumps that are itchy—known as urticaria pigmentosa) and gastrointestinal mucosa involvement. In adults, the spleen and liver are also often involved. The ulcer she developed is from histamine-mediated hypersecretion of gastric acid. You can confirm the diagnosis by measuring urine for histamine metabolites or by measuring increased levels of serum histamine or mast cell-derived neutral protease tryptase. Common variable immunodeficiency is characterized by recurrent sinopulmonary infections, not symptoms of histamine release. Anaphylaxis to several agents might cause some of her symptoms, but would not result in persistent skin lesions or a duodenal ulcer. Hereditary angioedema manifests with repeated episodes of swelling, not with discrete urticarial lesions or persistent rash. Urticaria is not the best answer because, although the lesions of urticaria pigmentosa do have the appearance of hives when irritated, routine urticaria would not be expected to result in the other systemic symptoms described in this patient.

Board Testing Point: Recognize the clinical features of systemic mastocytosis.

498. Answer: B

Answer: Serum immunoglobulins.
He most likely has immunoglobulin A deficiency. IgA serves as the first line of defense against infections of the respiratory tract, as well as infections of the GI and GU tracts. IgA deficiency is really fairly common! 1/600 individuals of European ancestry will have the deficiency. People with IgA deficiency are usually healthy, but they may have frequent episodes of upper respiratory tract infections, bronchiectasis, and chronic diarrhea. They are also more prone to allergies, asthma, and other autoimmune disorders. This patient does not have risk factors for HIV infection, and HIV infection would not account for his increased frequency of childhood infections. SPEP might help identify excess immunoglobulins, but not deficiency of them. Cold agglutinins are IgM antibodies that agglutinate red blood cells and are seen in various infections, autoimmune disorders, and lymphoma. They may also occur as a primary autoimmune disease. However, especially in the absence of symptoms suggestive of lymphoma, one would not expect them to be associated with frequent upper airway infections. CH50 is used to evaluate the function of the classical pathway of complement. Frequent upper airway infections are not characteristic of complement deficiencies.

Board Testing Point: Recognize clinical features of immunoglobulin A deficiency.

499. Answer: B

Answer: Acute hypersensitivity pneumonitis.
Given the temporal relationship between the exposure to the mice, the nonspecific infiltrates, and the restrictive pulmonary physiology, acute hypersensitivity pneumonitis is the most likely diagnosis. Acute hypersensitivity pneumonitis is characterized by an influenza-like illness and respiratory symptoms after exposure to the offending antigen. In this case, the antigen is from proteins found in mice urine, serum, and/or pelt. The best therapy is to remove the patient from the environment, because chronic exposure could lead to a subacute or chronic form of this disease with potentially serious physiologic consequences. The clue to the diagnosis is that the symptoms improve when the patient is away from work.

Granulomatosis with polyangiitis is characterized by the clinical triad of upper airway involvement, lower respiratory tract involvement, and glomerulonephritis. Both acute bronchitis and leptospirosis can result in influenza-like symptoms. However, a history of symptoms improving when the patient is away from work argues against granulomatosis, acute bronchitis, and leptospirosis. Although there is a casual relationship between workplace exposure and occupational asthma, one would not expect to find pulmonary infiltrates with asthma. Furthermore, the presence of influenza-like symptoms (stuffy nose, cough, fever, and chills) and restrictive lung pathology argues against occupational asthma.

Board Testing Point: Recognize the clinical features of acute hypersensitivity pneumonitis.

500. Answer: D

Answer: Metered dose albuterol inhaler before she exercises.
Exercise-induced bronchoconstriction (EIB) is defined as acute airway narrowing that occurs as a result of vigorous exercise. Inhaled short-acting beta-agonists (such as albuterol) are the single most effective agents to protect against EIB. Albuterol administered 5–20 minutes before exercise is effective for 2–4 hours in preventing EIB when used intermittently. Use of glucocorticosteroids (either oral or inhaled) prior to exercise is not effective in protecting against EIB. **Daily** inhaled corticosteroids (ICS) may be considered for patients with EIB who continue to have symptoms despite using inhaled albuterol before exercise, or who required daily or more frequent use of albuterol prior to exercise. Theophylline is not recommened for the treatment of EIB. Of note, warm-up exercises before planned exercise are also recommended to prevent EIB.

Board Testing Point: Recognize the clinical features of exercise-induced bronchoconstriction and that prophylactic albuterol inhaler before exercise will prevent attacks.

501. Answer: D

Answer: Skin biopsy.
The combination of residual skin lesions, arthralgias, and elevated ESR are not consistent with hereditary angioedema or most urticarial diseases. It is much more likely due to urticarial vasculitis, which could be confirmed by skin biopsy. Chronic urticaria is rarely allergic in nature; therefore, allergy skin testing and IgE levels are not likely to be helpful. C1 esterase inhibitor activity level would be useful in hereditary angioedema, but not in this entity. The patch test would be helpful in diagnosing contact dermatitis.

Board Testing Point: Recognize the clinical features of urticarial vasculitis.

502. Answer: B

Answer: Monthly intravenous immunoglobulin.
This patient's presentation is most consistent with common variable immunodeficiency (CVID). B cells can recognize antigen and multiply, but fail to differentiate to the immunoglobulin-secreting stage. Nodular lymphoid hyperplasia and splenomegaly are commonly found in these patients. Recurrent *Giardia* infections may also occur. These patients have low IgG, IgA, and frequently IgM. The therapy for common variable immunodeficiency is replacement of immunoglobulin—mainly immunoglobulin G—with IV or subcutaneous immunoglobulin replacement. Corticosteroids do not have a role in improving the hypogamaglobulinemia. Splenectomy has not been shown to play a role in treatment in the absence of co-morbid hematologic disease. Bone marrow transplantation also has not been shown to be helpful in CVID. Infusions of IgG, not IgA, are the mainstay of treatment.

Board Testing Point: Recognize the clinical features of common variable immunodeficiency, and know appropriate treatment.

503. Answer: C

Answer: Equine antithymocyte globulin.
The patient has developed serum sickness from equine antithymocyte globulin. All of his features are classic for a severe reaction to an agent like this one. Usually it occurs 1–3 weeks after receiving the therapy. The Boards are also likely to ask this question in reference to a snake bite in a patient who receives anti-venom. Serum sickness is a hypersensitivity reaction that occurs when an antibody reacts with a target antigen to form immune complexes. The immune complexes precipitate in small blood vessels and activate complement with subsequent small vessel inflammation and necrosis. Serum sickness is usually self-limited after withdrawal of the offending drug and the antigen is cleared. Occasionally, corticosteroids are given. Of the available choices, equine entithymocyte globulin is the most likely cause of serum sickness.

Board Testing Point: Recognize the clinical features of serum sickness.

504. Answer: E

Answer: By causing an IgE-mediated reaction against proteins in the bee venom.
Anaphylaxis due to bee stings, foods, and heterologous serum (such as tetanus antitoxin) is likely due to an IgE-mediated reaction against the offending protein. IgA does not play a role in immediate hypersensitivity. Anaphylaxis due to penicillin and other antibiotics is due to IgE recognition of protein-hapten conjugants. In contrast, radiocontrast media directly activates mast cells and basophils to release the mediators of anaphylaxis. Finally, deficiency of C1 esterase results in hereditary angioedema, not anaphylaxis.

Board Testing Point: Know the mechanism for a bee sting to cause anaphylaxis.

505. Answer: D

Answer: She had IgE recognition of protein-hapten conjugants.
Anaphylaxis due to penicillin and other antibiotics is due to IgE recognition of protein-hapten conjugants. Anaphylaxis due to bee stings, foods, and heterologous serum (such as tetanus antitoxin) is likely due to an IgE-mediated reaction against the offending protein. In contrast, radiocontrast media directly activates these cells to release the mediators of anaphylaxis. Finally, dialysis induces anaphylaxis with complement activation.

Board Testing Point: Recognize the mechanism for anaphylaxis to penicillin.

---

506. Answer: A

Answer: Henoch-Schönlein purpura.
He has the classic findings of purpura that are confined to the buttocks and lower extremities. Additionally, he has signs of gastrointestinal involvement as well as glomerulonephritis. The classic triad of Henoch-Schönlein purpura (HSP) are purpura, arthritis, and abdominal pain. HSP is a small vessel vasculitis characterized by deposition of IgA immune complexes. Most of the time HSP is self-limiting, but occasionally it can progress to a chronic form. Leukemia can present with purpura but typically has abnormalities on CBC. Job syndrome (Hyper-IgE syndrome) is characterized by recurrent infections and markedly elevated immunoglobulin E.

Board Testing Point: Recognize the clinical features of Henoch-Schönlein purpura.

---

507. Answer: D

Answer: T cells lack readily detectable immunoglobulin of <u>any</u> class on their membranes.
Remember that detectable immunoglobulins are found on B cells.

Board Testing Point: Remember that immunoglobulin is found only on B cells.

---

508. Answer: E

Answer: All of the statements are true.
IgA is found mainly at mucosal surfaces of the respiratory, gastrointestinal, and genitourinary tracts where it fights infection. It is produced in large quantities daily and mostly stays in body secretions rather than circulating in the blood. It exists as 2 subclasses: IgA1 and IgA2. Lastly, there is evidence that it can interfere with microbial binding to epithelial cell surfaces as a way to prevent infections.

Board Testing Point: Know the characteristics of immunoglobulin A.

---

509. Answer: A

Answer: Isolated IgA deficiency.
Isolated IgA deficiency is the most common immunodeficiency and has an incidence between 1:600 and 1:800. People with this disorder have a normal or reduced number of B cells with surface IgA, but have an overabundance of immature cells that express both IgA and IgM. Because they do not mature normally into IgA-secreting plasma cells, there is a reduced amount of serum as well as secretory IgA. About 30–40% of people with IgA deficiency have antibodies to IgA; therefore, if they are exposed to IgA (like in blood products or IVIG), they will experience anaphylaxis. Terminal complement deficiency results in inability to form the membrane attack complex and susceptibility to neisserial infections. Systemic mastocytosis does not lead to increased infections. IgG deficiency commonly leads to severe sinopulmonary infections. IgD deficiency does not predispose to increased infections.

Board Testing Point: Recognize the clinical features of isolated IgA deficiency.

510. Answer: C

Answer: Most immune complexes are removed by the mononuclear phagocyte (reticuloendothelial) system.
Deposition of the immune complexes in tissues other than the reticuloendothelial system is what results in signs and symptoms of immune-complex disease. It appears that persistence of complexes is required for the development of renal disease. Immune complex-mediated vascular damage can lead to cutaneous necrotizing vasculitis.

Board Testing Point: Know that immune complexes are removed by the mononuclear phagocyte (reticuloendothelial) system.

511. Answer: A

Answer: Mature red blood cells.
All nucleated cells of the body express Class I HLA antigens. Remember that Class I HLA antigens are encoded at the A, B, and C loci of the human major histocompatibility complex on chromosome 6. The Class I HLA antigens are useful in predicting results for organ transplants.

Board Testing Point: Recognize that mature red blood cells do not express Class I HLA antigens.

512. Answer: B

Answer: Decongestants/nasal irrigation.
This patient presents with a 5-day history of rhinorrhea, sore throat, and facial pain. She is afebrile with swollen nasal turbinates on exam. Her symptom complex is most consistent with the common cold. The CDC campaign to limit antibiotic use advises to wait 7–10 days before considering treatment with antibiotics for "sinusitis" for facial pain/persistent congestion. The yellow discharge does not increase the likelihood of a bacterial infection. The best treatment would be to begin saline nasal irrigation and topical decongestants for several days **without** antibiotic treatment.

Board Testing Point: Recognize that the diagnosis of bacterial sinusitis generally requires 7–10 days of symptoms before initiating antibiotic therapy.

513. Answer: D

Answer: C1 esterase inhibitor.
The classic pathway of complement activation is initiated by antibody-antigen interaction. The first complement component (C1, a complex composed of 3 proteins) binds to immune complexes with activation mediated by C1q. Active C1 then initiates the cleavage and concomitant activation of components C4 and C2. The activated C1 is destroyed by a plasma protease inhibitor known as C1 esterase inhibitor. Patients with deficiencies of C1 esterase inhibitor may develop angioedema, which can lead to death if it involves the larynx or other parts of the respiratory tract. T-cell receptor alpha chain deficiency is reported to cause increase risk of infection and autoimmune complications, not episodic swelling. Low levels of C5a, IgE, and cyclooxygenase likewise are not associated with swelling.

Board Testing Point: Recognize the clinical features of angioedema and its association with C1 esterase inhibitor deficiency.

---

514. Answer: E

Answer: It is associated with low IgM.
Wiskott-Aldrich syndrome is an X-linked disorder characterized by eczema, thrombocytopenia, and recurrent infections. Usually these patients have **high levels** of IgA and IgE. They are at increased risk for infection, and they can be treated successfully with bone marrow transplantation.

Board Testing Point: Recognize clinical features of Wiskott-Aldrich syndrome.

---

515. Answer: A

Answer: Give epinephrine 0.3 mg to 0.5 mg IM.
Remember that IV steroids are not acutely effective, and trials have shown no real benefit. Subcutaneous epinephrine is no longer recommended because the absorption is haphazard; IM administration is the preferred method and provides more rapid plasma and tissue concentrations. Beta-blockade would be a disaster! It would blunt the effect of your epinephrine also! If she had bronchospasm, you would give albuterol inhalation.

Board Testing Point: Know how to treat anaphylaxis.

---

516. Answer: A

Answer: Kawasaki disease.
She has all of the classic findings: She has fever, which is a requirement, and she has:

- Conjunctivitis
- Erythematous mouth and pharynx, strawberry tongue, and red, cracked lips
- Generalized rash
- Changes to the peripheral extremities, consisting of induration of the hands and feet with red palms and soles
- Unilateral cervical lymph node enlarged to more than 1.5 cm in diameter

Patients must have fever and at least 4 of the 5 findings for diagnosis. If there are fewer than 4 classic findings, then a diagnosis of atypical Kawasaki's should be considered. Treatment is with IVIG 2 g/kg x 1 time dose over 12–14 hours and aspirin in high doses initially, followed by low-maintenance doses. Usually, Kawasaki's appears in children under the age of 5; however, cases in teenagers have been reported.

Board Testing Point: Recognize the clinical features of Kawasaki disease (although rare in teens, it can occur).

517. Answer: D

Answer: Aspirin.
All NSAIDs inhibit the synthesis of prostaglandins via binding to cyclooxygenase. However, aspirin is the **only** agent that binds irreversibly. This is likely why aspirin is the only NSAID that inhibits platelets—platelets cannot manufacture new cyclooxygenase! Therefore, remember to stop aspirin 7–10 days before elective surgical procedures where bleeding cannot be tolerated (eye, neurosurgery, etc.).

Board Testing Point: Recognize that aspirin irreversibly binds to cyclooxygenase.

DERMATOLOGY

518. Answer: B

Answer: Hepatitis C.
Hepatitis C is frequently found in association with PCT. In addition to vesicles of the skin, there can also be increased pigmentation, increased fragility, milia formation, and increased facial hair. Patients with PCT also have an increased incidence of liver cirrhosis and liver cancer. PCT due to HCV resolves with treatment of hepatitis C. Acanthosis nigricans, hepatitis B, and paraneoplastic pemphigus are not associated with PCT.

Board Testing Point: Recognize the clinical association of hepatitis C with porphyria cutanea tarda.

519. Answer: C

Answer: Glucagonoma syndrome.
Erosions of the skin and mucous membranes characterize the glucagonoma syndrome. The lesions are referred to as necrolytic migratory erythema. Patients may also have glossitis, weight loss, hyperglycemia, and decreased plasma amino acids. Sweet syndrome (acute febrile neutrophilic dermatosis) presents with vesicular-like papules, fever, and leukocytosis. Carcinoid syndrome is characterized by flushing of the skin, and primary amyloidosis usually presents with pinch purpura. When glucagonoma syndrome is diagnosed, it is important to rule out a zinc or magnesium deficiency because they can have a similar presentation. Patients with glucagonoma syndrome have an alpha cell tumor of the pancreas, and the sooner it is found and treated, the better the prognosis.

Board Testing Point: Recognize the clinical features of glucagonoma syndrome.

520. Answer: C

Answer: Refer her for excisional biopsy of the lesion.
Superficial spreading melanoma is the most common type of melanoma, and comprises 70 percent of all melanomas. It is found predominantly in young people who burn rather than tan. The favored location is on the back of the legs of women and on the backs of men. When such a lesion is identified, referral is indicated for simple excision and histological evaluation. Based on the depth of invasion, re-excision margins are decided, and the patient's prognosis is determined. A punch biopsy of the brown area will show melanocytes in the epidermis, which may or may not be malignant and could result in an inaccurate diagnosis. Likewise, liquid nitrogen will remove only the superficial portion of the tumor, leaving the dermal portion to proliferate and metastasize. Whenever a melanoma is suspected, intervention is indicated because malignant melanoma is a life-threatening disease.

Board Testing Point: Recognize the clinical features of melanoma, and know that excisional biopsy is the best diagnostic and potentially therapeutic procedure.

521. Answer: E

Answer: Cutaneous candidal infection.
Typically, these infections occur at sites that are chronically wet and macerated, such as an intertriginous area that requires frequent water exposure (like in the case of this nurse). Treatment would involve a topical agent such as topical clotrimazole. Acanthosis nigricans is hyperpigmented skin with a thickened, velvety appearance, noticed mostly in the skin folds and commonly seen in obese patients. Plaques psoriasis manifests as erythematous skin lesions with distinctive silvery scales. It is usually symmetric and occurs on extensor surfaces of the knees and elbows, the sacral area, and the scalp. The history and lesions described would not be typical of human papilloma virus (warts) or cutaneous bacterial infection.

Board Testing Point: Recognize the clinical features of cutaneous candidal infection and its epidemiological features.

522. Answer: C

Answer: Topical tretinoin.
The diagnosis of acne is established when 3 of the 6 lesions of acne are present. The lesions of acne are papules, pustules, open and closed comedones, ice pick scars, hyperpigmented macules, and cystic lesions. If, as in this patient, the majority of the lesions are noninflammatory, topical retinoids are the treatment of choice because of their keratolytic effect. The other choices listed are not keratolytic and thus would be less effective for the patient described.

Board Testing Point: Topical retinoids are the drug of choice for mild noninflammatory acne.

523. Answer: B

Answer: Topical steroids.
Topical steroids are the mainstay of therapy of treatment for atopic skin. However, they are not recommended for prolonged use on the face or intertriginous areas because they can cause striae, atrophy, telangiectasias, pigmentary changes, and acneiform skin eruptions.Tacrolimus (Protopic®) and pimecrolimus (Elidel®) are topical immunosuppressants (calcineurin inhibitors) that are effective alternatives to topical corticosteroids. Since these don't cause skin atrophy, they are especially good for facial lesions. There is a potential risk of skin cancer or T-cell lymphoma, so these agents are 2nd line for intermittent treatment of atopic dermatitis. These agents should be avoided in HIV+ patients or anyone with a weakened immune system. Currently, most prescribers counsel patients about this risk, but the risk of severe local side effects from topical steroids outweighs the risk of calcineurin inhibitors for lesions involving the face. Lubrication alone would not be expected to produce local side effects.

Board Testing Point: Recognize that topical steroids should not be used for prolonged periods of time on the face or intertriginious areas. Topical calcineurin inhibitors are an effective alternative that do not cause striae, atrophy, and telangiectasias.

524. Answer: D

Answer: Dermatomyositis and cancer.
The classic presentation of dermatomyositis is a heliotrope rash about the eyes, proximal muscle weakness, erythema and telangiectasia of the cuticles, and palmar erythema. It is thought that the papules over the joints (Gottron papules) are pathognomonic of dermatomyositis. Patients over 50 years of age are at risk for their dermatomyositis being associated with internal malignancy. The weight loss associated with the typical findings of dermatomyositis makes this the most likely diagnosis.

Board Testing Point: Recognize that in older patients, dermatomyositis may be a paraneoplastic phenomenon. (GU/ovarian, GI, lung, and lymphoma are most common.) All patients diagnosed with dermatomyositis should be offered age-appropriate cancer screening.

---

525. Answer: C

Answer: Erythema nodosum.
In addition to sarcoidosis, erythema nodosum can be associated with streptococcal infections, inflammatory bowel disease, tuberculosis, and drug allergy. The association of erythema nodosum, arthritis, anterior uveitis, and hilar adenopathy due to sarcoidosis is termed Löfgren syndrome, and is usually associated with a good prognosis. Although the classic Löfgren syndrome is a tetrad, the term is commonly applied when a patient presents with only sarcoidosis and erythema nodosum. The lack of appropriate history and the appearance of the biopsy exclude the other diagnoses. Erythema nodosum can be treated with nonsteroidal antiinflammatory drugs, topical or systemic steroids, or immunosuppressive agents.

Board Testing Point: Recognize Löfgren syndrome and the other entities associated with erythema nodosum.

---

526. Answer: A

Answer: Impetigo vulgaris.
The trauma caused by scratching has broken the skin and permitted bacterial invasion and secondary infection. Most community-acquired skin infections are due to streptococcal or staphylococcal species. Impetigo vulgaris is most often caused by *Staphylococci*. Erythema nodosum most often presents as tender nodules on the pre-tibial surfaces of the legs.The clinical manifestations of acne vulgaris are open ("blackheads") and closed ("whiteheads") comedones, papules, pustules, and cystic lesions. In general, drug eruptions most commonly start on the chest, abdomen, or the back.

Board Testing Point: Recognize the clinical features of impetigo vulgaris.

---

527. Answer: D

Answer: Bullous pemphigoid.
Bullous pemphigoid is an autoimmune blistering disease of the elderly that may begin and remain on the legs for a number of years before involving the rest of the skin. It is pruritic in nature and can involve the mucosa. While occurring on normal or erythematous skin, the bullae are intact and give a negative Nikolsky sign. Pemphigus vulagaris manifests as loose bullae that peel off and leave denuded skin. Nikosky sign is positive in pemphigus vulgaris. Treatment of both bullous pemphigoid and pemphigus vulgaris consist of topical steroids alone in localized disease and systemic steroids in more severe or widespread disease. Dermatitis herpetiformis is a skin disease where very pruritic vesicular lesions appear, usually on the extensor surfaces and mid to lower back, caused by IgA deposition in the dermal papillary tips. Given the extreme pruritus, intact vesicles are often not apparent. It is associated with celiac disease. Erythema multiforme consists of well-defined lesions varying from annular to targetoid. Palms and soles are frequently involved, and mucous membranes may be affected. The "target" lesions are pathognomonic for erythema multiforme, and it is most commonly caused by herpes simplex viral infection.

Board Testing Point: Recognize the clinical features of bullous pemphigoid.

528. Answer: A

Answer: Herpetic infections.
Exfoliative dermatitis (erythroderma) is not associated with herpes simplex or herpes zoster. It is frequently seen as an allergic reaction to such drugs as sulfonamides, anti-malarials, penicillin, phenytoin, and barbiturates. It has also been associated with psoriasis, atopic dermatitis, or malignancy (especially cutaneous T-cell lymphoma). No matter what the etiology, the skin biopsy is often nonspecific. The course and prognosis of exfoliative dermatitis is related to the course of the underlying process. Drug-induced exfoliative dermatitis has the best prognosis while those associated with malignancy have the highest mortality.

Board Testing Point: Recognize that exfoliative dermatitis is associated with drugs, atopic dermatitis, psoriasis, and malignancy.

529. Answer: D

Answer: Doxycycline.
This patient develops a rash after taking an antibiotic while on vacation in Hawaii. The distribution of the rash is strongly suggestive of a photosensitivity reaction. The tetracyclines have a known increased risk of phototoxicity. Amoxicillin/clavulanate, cefixime, and nitrofurantoin do not cause phototoxic reactions. Other agents that commonly cause phototoxicity include furosemide, sulfonamides, amiodarone, thiazides, and phenothiazines.

Board Testing Point: Know that doxycycline, fluoroquinolones, furosemide, and amiodarone are common causes of phototoxicity.

530. Answer: B

Answer: Dyshidrotic eczema.
Hand dermatitis is quite common in individuals who wash their hands frequently, and this dishwasher has a common variant of this type of eczema. The finding of highly pruritic vesicles on the sides of the fingers is helpful in making this diagnosis. Lichen planus is a disorder with papulosquamous pruritic lesions that have a purplish hue. Lichen planus also causes ulceration and lace-like patches (Wickham striae). Herpes simplex (oral-genital) and zoster (dermatomal) would present as a group of vesicles on an erythematous base. Atopic dermatitis would be more likely if she had a history of asthma or disease during childhood.

Board Testing Point: Recognize the clinical features of dyshidrotic eczema.

531. Answer: A

Answer: Osler-Rendu-Weber disease.
Osler-Weber-Rendu syndrome, or hereditary hemorrhagic telangiectasis, is an autosomal dominant disorder manifested by mucocutaneous telangiectases and arteriovenous malformations. Patients commonly present with epistaxis or gastrointestinal bleeding. CREST features include calcinosis cutis (small tender nodules on the fingers), Raynaud syndrome, esophageal dysmotility, sclerodactyly of the fingers, and telangiectasias. Anti-centromere antibody (ACA) is specific for limited SSc and is seen in about 50% of patients. It is a form of limited scleroderma. Malar (or butterfly) rash occurs in about half of acute SLE patients and rarely occurs in patients without systemic symptoms. Classically, this rash involves both cheeks and extends across the bridge of the nose, sparing the nasolabial fold and often occurs after sunlight exposure (photosensitive).

Board Testing Point: Recognize the clinical features of Osler-Rendu-Weber disease.

532. Answer: D

Answer: Syphilis.
He has a classic rash of secondary syphilis. The palm and sole involvement is the "hallmark" for this disease. The painless chancre lesion is commonly on the penis; but depending upon sexual practices, it can be on the pharynx or anus. Dermatomyositis is associated with a periorbital heliotrope rash and Gottron's papules over the knuckles. SLE is associated with malar (or butterfly) rash. Classically, this rash involves both cheeks and extends across the bridge of the nose, sparing the nasolabial fold. Common rashes associated with HIV include seborrheic dermatitis, kaposi sarcoma, oral candidiasis ("thrush"), and oral hairy leukoplakia. Bacterial endocarditis is associated with Osler nodes (raised and painful) and Janeway lesions (flat and painless) that typically occur on the hands and feet.

Board Testing Point: Recognize the clinical features of secondary syphilis.

533. Answer: C

Answer: Folate deficiency.
He has vitiligo, an autoimmune disease that causes destruction of melanocytes resulting in depigmentation. It may rarely be associated with other autoimmune diseases, particularly as part of a polyglandular autoimmune deficiency syndrome. All of the conditions listed except for folate are associated with vitiligo. Anytime you see a patient with vitiligo, think of these possibilities and screen appropriately!

Board Testing Point: Recognize vitiligo and its associated disease processes.

534. Answer: A

Answer: Amoxicillin-clavulanate.
This patient has experienced a cat bite. Animal bites carry the risk of infection from a wide variety of pathogens, including skin flora such as *Staphylococcus* and *Streptococcus*. In addition, bites from animals or humans also carry increased risk of infections with anaerobes. Cat and dog oral flora frequently includes *Pasteurella species* that can cause potentially serious infection.

Antimicrobial therapy is indicated for prophylaxis after a bite, even in the absence of infection, and should cover all of the above mentioned pathogens. Amoxicillin-clavulanate would cover those and is recommended 1st line therapy. Neither cephalexin nor erythromycin has activity against *Pasteurella*. Moxifloxacin does have coverage against *Pasteurella* but should be combined with clindamycin in order to provide adequate anaerobic coverage. Clindamycin with erythromycin does not have coverage for *Pasteurella*.

Board Testing Point: Identify appropriate prophylaxis treatment of *Pasteurella species* in the management of animal bites.

535. Answer: B

Answer: Cephalexin.
Diffuse cellulitis with no portal of entry, purulent drainage, or exudate and no associated abscess is known as "non-purulent" cellulitis. It is most commonly caused by streptococcal species and should be managed with empiric therapy for infection due to beta-hemolytic streptococci and MSSA; i.e., coverage of MRSA is not warranted. So, cephalexin is the correct choice.

Vancomycin is not appropriate outpatient management for uncomplicated cellulitis. Neither doxycycline nor trimethoprim/sulfamethoxazole (TMP/SMX) would adequately cover for streptococci unless they are used in combination with an antistreptococcal agent (e.g., amoxicillin).

Know that empiric therapy is a starting point and can be changed by regional considerations; e.g., if your area has a high incidence of MRSA, you take that into account also.

Board Testing Point: Know antibiotic therapy for nonpurulent cellulitis.

GENERAL INTERNAL MEDICINE

536. Answer: B

Answer: Methanol.
Methanol and ethylene glycol are the only agents that will potentially give you both a metabolic and an osmotic gap.

Board Testing Point: Recognize that methanol and ethylene glycol are associated with both a metabolic and osmotic gap.

537. Answer: D

Answer: 12.5%.
To calculate positive predictive value, divide true positives by (true positives + false positives). In this case:

25 / (25 + 175) = 12.5%

Board Testing Point: Understand how to calculate positive predictive value.

538. Answer: A

Answer: 5.
Number of people needed to treat to prevent 1 bad outcome is based on 1/(absolute risk reduction) = 1/(the rate in the placebo group minus the rate in treatment group).

In our example: 1 / (20/50 – 10/50) = 1 / (0.4 – 0.2) = 1 / (0.2) = 5

Board Testing Point: Know how to calculate the number needed to treat.

539. Answer: D

Answer: The nephew's request to discontinue IVF and antibiotics is within his capacity to act as the patient's durable power of attorney for health care.
If someone has a durable power of attorney for health care—that person rules if the patient cannot make decisions for herself.

Board Testing Point: Recognize that a durable power of attorney for medical affairs (health care) has the legal right to make decisions and supersedes family members.

540. Answer: B

Answer: Treat with antibiotics because the patient has a life-threatening condition.
This patient has a life-threatening condition (meningitis) that is likely affecting the patient's ability to make an informed decision. The patient has not refused medical care and has agreed to an invasive procedure (LP) but does not want antibiotics. You are not given information that the patient has a long-standing stance against medication. The patient is somnolent and agitated when aroused, which is a change in baseline mental functioning. Because the patient has not demonstrated competency and is incapacitated by an acute illness, it is appropriate as the physician to intervene in the best interest of the patient. If a family member were present, then discussing it with him/her would be appropriate. A roommate has less decision-making authority in this case than the physician. Court orders are not practical in urgent situations like meningitis.

Board Testing Point: Recognize that if a patient is incapable of making a rational medical decision in a life-threatening condition, a physician may determine what is the best possible decision if no family member is available to assist in the decision-making process.

541. Answer: C

Answer: Detrusor overactivity.
This patient has typical symptoms of urge incontinence; that is, she gets the message to urinate but is unable to make it to the toilet in time. Urge incontinence is due to detrusor overactivity. None of the medications she is on cause incontinence. Common medications that can lead to incontinence are diuretics and anticholinergic medications.

Board Testing Point: Recognize the clinical features of urge incontinence and the common mechanism for it.

542. Answer: A

Answer: Mammogram, Pap smear, and colonoscopy.
This patient has not had any medical care or screening for at least 12 years. She should have Pap smear testing because she has not been screened for many years (if ever). It is appropriate not to do Pap testing in patients 65 or older if they are low-risk (no new sexual partners and multiple prior normal Pap smears). She should have a mammogram and colonoscopy (or other colon screening test) according to USPSTF and ACS guidelines. Clinical breast examination is controversial, while CBC is rarely, if ever, a screening test.

Board Testing Point: Recognize the recommended screening tests for women at age 65 (the Medicare visit).

543. Answer: C

Answer: After the patient responds to emergent therapy, she may develop profound amnesic psychosis.
Wernicke encephalopathy is a consequence of thiamine (vitamin B_1) deficiency. It is most commonly seen in chronic alcoholics; however, well-documented cases have occurred in those without any alcohol intake. The classic triad (ophthalmoplegia, ataxia, and encephalopathy) is rare. **Always** administer thiamine before glucose! Glucose in the absence of thiamine will worsen the disease! Thiamine administration will relieve the ocular palsies within hours. The ataxia and encephalopathy will resolve more slowly; but frequently, the encephalopathy will leave a marked defect in memory and learning, known as Korsakoff psychosis. The major sites of brain involvement include the thalamus, hypothalamus, midbrain, floor of the 4th ventricle, and the cerebellar vermis.

Board Testing Point: Recognize the clinical features of Wernicke encephalopathy.

544. Answer: A

Answer: Benazepril/lithium interaction.
This patient presents with symptoms consistent with lithium toxicity (diarrhea, nausea, vomiting, and ataxia; on exam, he has fasciculations, cogwheel rigidity, and hyperreflexia). He was recently started on benazepril for hypertension. All ACE inhibitors inhibit renal excretion of lithium. Cimetidine and carbamazepine do not affect lithium levels.

Board Testing Point: Recognize the drug-drug interaction of benazepril and lithium.

545. Answer: A

Answer: Emergent referral to an ophthalmologist for gonioscopy.
This technique involves using a special lens for the slit lamp, which allows the ophthalmologist to visualize the angle and diagnose angle closure. The patient has acute angle-closure glaucoma. This has resulted in the obstruction of outflow from the aqueous humor at the iris. The buildup of intraocular pressure can be measured and requires urgent treatment with hyperosmotic agents. Permanent treatment will require peripheral iridotomy.

Board Testing Point: Recognize the clinical features of acute angle-closure glaucoma and the need for emergent ophthalmologic referral.

546. Answer: B

Answer: HIV retinopathy.
This patient with HIV presents without visual symptoms. On funduscopic exam, he has cotton wool spots without hemorrhage, suggesting HIV retinopathy. His high CD4 count effectively rules out CMV retinitis (almost always seen with CD4 count less than 50) and toxoplasmosis (rare above CD4 count of 100). *Cryptococcus* and *Cryptosporidia* rarely ever cause retinal lesions.

Board Testing Point: Recognize that opportunistic eye diseases occur in patients with HIV who have low CD4 counts (CMV is the most commonly asked about if the CD4 count is low; otherwise, HIV retinopathy is more likely).

547. Answer: E

Answer: Methyldopa.
This woman has signs and symptoms of preeclampsia with increased BP and edema. She does not have headache or neurologic findings. She needs to be treated with an antihypertensive agent. In pregnancy, there is good data to show what **not** to use: ACE inhibitors and nitroprusside should not be used. Other drugs to avoid include isotretinoin, benzodiazepines, quinolones, tetracyclines, and warfarin. Generally, you would avoid diuretics to prevent dehydration and electrolyte disturbances, and minoxidil is not recommended in pregnancy. Labetalol has become a drug of choice in many centers for treatment of hypertension as well, although the Boards still tend to list methyldopa as the most common drug (they would not make you pick between methyldopa and labetalol).

Board Testing Point: Recognize that for treatment of hypertension in pregnancy, the best initial choice is likely to be either methyldopa or labetalol.

548. Answer: D

Answer: Cerumen impaction.
This patient has noticed decreased hearing in his right ear. He has risk factors for hearing loss, including recent treatment with aminoglycosides. The results of the Rinne test and Weber test are diagnostic in this case. The Rinne test shows air conduction louder than bone conduction in the left ear and bone conduction louder than air conduction in the right ear (symptomatic ear). This is consistent with a conductive hearing loss in his right ear. The Weber test confirms this by lateralizing to the ear with the conductive hearing loss. Aminoglycoside toxicity would cause a sensory hearing loss, as would acoustic neuroma and Ménière disease and cochlear osteosclerosis. Unilateral cerumen impaction would cause a conductive hearing loss on the side of the impaction.

Board Testing Point: Recognize how to use the Rinne and Weber tests for determining what type of hearing abnormality is present.

549. Answer: D

Answer: Cyclosporine.
Cyclosporine is one of the drugs that will increase serum uric acid. This man has **gout**. This is a drug interaction question! Other drugs that will increase serum uric acid include diuretics, niacin, and ethambutol/pyrazinamide.

Board Testing Point: Recognize the side effects of cyclosporine.

550. Answer: B

Answer: Ciprofloxacin.
Common photosensitivity medications include tetracyclines, sulfonamides, hydrochlorothiazide, phenothiazines, griseofulvin, and other quinolones. From highest risk to lowest risk of the quinolones:

1) Sparfloxacin (no longer available in U.S.)
2) Lomefloxacin (no longer available in U.S.)
3) Nalidixic acid (no longer available in U.S.)
4) Enoxacin (no longer available in U.S.)
5) Ciprofloxacin
6) Norfloxacin
7) Levofloxacin
8) Trovafloxacin (no longer available in U.S., except for extreme circumstances)

Board Testing Point: In case an older question like this appears on the Boards, recognize that quinolones have a higher risk of photosensitivity.

551. Answer: C

Answer: "Get up and go" test.
When evaluating falls in the elderly, one should include a number of factors, such as medical conditions, vision and hearing, vestibular function, cognitive impairment, medications, and environmental conditions such as the safety of the living quarters. On physical examination, muscle strength and coordination are extremely important, and specifically testing for integrated musculoskeletal function is crucial. In the elderly, the "get up and go" test is a reliable and valid test for quantifying functional mobility and has been recognized as the best functional test of integrated strength and function in the elderly, and may also be useful in following clinical change over time.

Board Testing Point: Understand functional testing in the elderly.

552. Answer: A

Answer: Amitriptyline.
Serum levels are not helpful in the management of tricyclic antidepressant overdoses!

Board Testing Point: Know that serum levels are not helpful in assessing tricyclic antidepressant overdoses.

553. Answer: B

Answer: 33.3%.
This question asks you to calculate the sensitivity of fecal occult blood testing in a defined patient population. To calculate sensitivity, divide the number of patients with a positive heme test who have cancer (true positives) by the number of all patients with colon cancer in the study (true positives **plus** false negatives). For this case, it would be 12 (the number of patients with heme-positive stool who have cancer) divided by (12 [those with heme-positive stool and cancer] + 24 [those with cancer who had heme-negative stool]):

$$12 / (12 + 24) = 12 / 36 = 1/3 = 33.3\%$$

Board Testing Point: Understand how to calculate sensitivity.

554. Answer: A

Answer: 98.9%.
To calculate negative predictive value, divide true negatives by (false negatives + true negatives).
In this case: 890 / (10 + 890) = 98.9%.

Board Testing Point: Know how to calculate negative predictive value.

555. Answer: C

Answer: No.
The key here is the 95% confidence interval. The interval –2.5 to 80.6 crosses 0. This indicates that the differences between the new treatment and the standard therapy were **not** statistically significant. The numbers can be quite deceiving—even with such a large increase in survival. One possibility is that the study had too few patients to really have any power to show a significant difference between the two groups.

Board Testing Point: Understand how to interpret 95% confidence intervals.

556. Answer: C

Answer: 71.4%.
To calculate sensitivity, divide true positives by (true positives + false negatives).
In this case: 25 / (25 + 10) = 25 / 35 = 71.4%

Board Testing Point: Know how to calculate sensitivity.

557. Answer: B

Answer: 83.6%.
To calculate specificity divide true negatives by (true negatives + false positives).
In this case: 890 / (890 + 175) = 890 / 1,065 = 83.6%

Board Testing Point: Know how to calculate specificity.

558. Answer: E

Answer: Do not give blood products.
This patient has stated her opinion against receiving blood products. This is confirmed by her husband. The overriding principle here is patient autonomy. She does not wish to receive blood products, and it is not appropriate for medical personnel to give blood products in such circumstances. If she were making a decision when she was not competent, then obtaining a representative for the patient would be appropriate.

Board Testing Point: Recognize the right of a competent patient to reject medical intervention based on religious convictions.

559. Answer: A

Answer: Do not intubate patient; keep him comfortable.
This patient has clearly stated his wishes to not be intubated in the event of worsening pulmonary disease. He was competent at the time of the decision, and by not intubating him, you are respecting his wishes. The children's desires do not supersede the patient's right to autonomy.

Board Testing Point: Recognize that a patient's wishes that have been clearly delineated outweigh family member wishes.

560. Answer: D

Answer: Terazosin.
This 76-year-old man has typical symptoms of prostatic obstruction. It is likely due to BPH. He has a normal PSA. Given his advanced age, he does not need an aggressive workup for prostate cancer. The best initial treatment for BPH would be terazosin. Finasteride is not as effective as terazosin and also takes longer to be effective. If he had increasing symptoms despite medical therapy, then consideration for surgery would be reasonable.

Board Testing Point: Recognize benign prostatic hypertrophy and the best initial therapy.

561. Answer: C

Answer: Vascular disease.
This elderly patient has erectile dysfunction but normal libido. Testosterone deficiency is common in elderly men, but when it causes erectile dysfunction it usually also causes decrease in libido. SSRIs can cause sexual side effects in about 30% of patients, but these are usually decrease in interest and delayed orgasm, not erectile dysfunction. This patient is on a lipid-lowering medication, making vascular disease more likely (risk factors of age and hyperlipidemia).

Board Testing Point: Recognize that vascular disease is a common cause of erectile dysfunction.

562. Answer: B

Answer: Intraurethral alprostadil (MUSE®).
This patient has erectile dysfunction with a normal libido. The normal libido would make testosterone deficiency less likely. Testosterone replacement would be inappropriate without documented low testosterone levels. He should not receive sildenafil (Viagra®, Revatio®) because he is taking daily nitrates. Nitrate use is a contraindication for the use of sildenafil. A penile implant would not be an appropriate initial therapy for erectile dysfunction. Even though intraurethral alprostadil is probably the patient's least favorite choice, it is the best choice of those listed.

Board Testing Point: Recognize that sildenafil (and similar agents) are contraindicated in patients receiving nitrate therapy.

563. Answer: D

Answer: Cholesterol.
The patient is 76 years old with Parkinson disease and coronary artery disease. Prostate cancer screening is controversial; however, the USPSTF categorically recommends **against** PSA testing in men ≥ 75. Complete blood cell count is not an approved screening test. Cholesterol testing would be appropriate, given his known CAD. Short-term and long-term benefits with cholesterol treatment have been demonstrated in patients with CAD, although the evidence is slightly less clear in patients age 75 or older.

Board Testing Point: Recognize that PSA testing is no longer recommended for men ≥ 75 years of age.

564. Answer: B

Answer: Pneumococcal, annual influenza, hep A series, Tdap.
Patients with HIV should receive an annual influenza vaccine and a pneumococcal vaccine every 6 years. This patient should also receive a hepatitis A series because of his hepatitis C infection (and the hepatitis A vaccine is universally recommended in the U.S. as well). Hepatitis A can cause fatal hepatitis in hep C-infected individuals. A tetanus vaccine is appropriate, because he has not had one in over 10 years; the new guidelines now recommend giving Tdap, with the pertussis component. He does not need a hepatitis B booster because he has serologic evidence of past hepatitis B infection.

Board Testing Point: Know appropriate immunizations for an HIV-infected man who has not had immunizations in > 10 years.

565. Answer: B

Answer: It can be a very effective treatment for bipolar affective disorder.
Lithium is not a drug of choice for most major depressive disorders. It has many drug-drug interactions, and the patient should be informed to notify all prescribers of medications that he is on lithium. Lithium intoxication manifests as depression of mental status. Hypothyroidism is a potential side effect of the drug because it inhibits secretion of thyroid hormone.

Board Testing Point: Know important clinical features of lithium.

566. Answer: A

Answer: Good premorbid functioning.
Premorbid functioning is the best indicator of good prognosis. All of the other factors listed are actually predictors of poor prognosis.

Board Testing Point: Recognize that good premorbid functioning is the best predictor of a good prognosis in the initial diagnosis of schizophrenia.

567. Answer: C

Answer: Antipsychotic medications and psychosocial treatment.

Board Testing Point: Recognize that combined antipsychotic medications and behavioral therapy are the best treatment for schizophrenia.

568. Answer: D

Answer: Diphenhydramine or benztropine immediately.
He is having an acute dystonic reaction. This usually occurs in the first hours or days of treatment. It is most common in younger men. The symptoms will improve rapidly with treatment.

Board Testing Point: Recognize acute dystonic reaction and how to treat it.

569. Answer: E

Answer: All of the statements are true.
Know this! Men **commit** suicide more often than women, **but** women **attempt** suicide more often than men. Additional risk factors on the Boards to look out for include history of alcohol or substance abuse, history of violence, prior psychiatric history, and recent major life change (separation, loss of job, etc.).

Board Testing Point: Know basic facts about suicide and suicide risk in the United States.

570. Answer: A

Answer: Voluntary hospitalization unless he refuses, then institute involuntary commitment.
This man has made out a plan of action and has considered it in the last 24 hours. He needs to be hospitalized for his own protection at this point. It is not pertinent that he is "okay" now. He has a past history of suicide attempt, and yesterday he was actually making a plan to proceed with another attempt.

Board Testing Point: Recognize the need for hospitalization (either voluntary or involuntary) in a patient with a confirmed plan for suicide.

571. Answer: E

Answer: All items listed are helpful clues.
Be wary of the elderly patient with many of these symptoms/findings: anxiety, insomnia, anhedonia, poor concentration. Particularly be aware of anhedonia (loss of pleasure from activities that usually bring pleasure).

Board Testing Point: Know important clues to look for in the diagnosis of depression.

572. Answer: C

Answer: Adjustment disorder with depressed mood.
Look for this when "a bad thing happens" on the Boards. The patient then cannot handle it well and feels malaise or a sense of things not right, etc. They generally do not meet the criteria for "full-blown" depression.

Board Testing Point: Know how to discern that a patient may have adjustment disorder with depressed mood due to a sad/uncomfortable life event.

573. Answer: B

Answer: SSRI.
SSRIs are the drugs of first choice for generalized anxiety disorder. Buspirone is an alternate agent for anxiety if an SSRI or SNRI is not effective. A benzodiazepine (e.g., clonazepam) could be used, but they are addictive and sedating. MAO inhibitors, haloperidol, and lithium are not effective nor approved for generalized anxiety disorder.

Board Testing Point: Recognize the clinical utility of an SSRI, SNRI, or buspirone in the treatment of generalized anxiety disorder.

574. Answer: E

Answer: Beta-amyloid protein.
On a neuropathological level, Alzheimer's is characterized by neurofibrillary tangles, which may contain an abnormally phosphorylated form of a microtubular protein, as well as spherical deposits known as senile plaques. These plaques are made up of beta-amyloid protein.

Board Testing Point: Recognize that beta-amyloid protein has a role in the development of Alzheimer's.

575. Answer: B

Answer: Paroxetine.
Before paroxetine, imipramine historically had been a good choice for panic disorder, which this woman has. The other agents listed are not effective for panic disorder.

Board Testing Point: Recognize that SSRIs are the best initial medical therapy for panic attack/disorders.

576. Answer: A

Answer: Reduce the dose of chlorpromazine.
This patient has tardive dyskinesia—manifested by his tongue-thrusting and lip-smacking gestures. Postural dystonia can also be part of this syndrome. The best thing to do is reduce the dose of medication. The problem with this, of course, is that he may have worsening of his thought disorder—so you have to watch for that. Akathisia, which he doesn't have, is characterized by obligatory movement of the extremities and motor restlessness—it may respond to treatment with beta-blockers. Also, some patients will respond to clozapine.

Board Testing Point: Recognize the clinical features and treatment for tardive dyskinesia.

577. Answer: D

Answer: Left inferior quadrantanopia.
Poor language comprehension, fluent speech output, paraphasic errors, and poor repetition are common in patients with Wernicke aphasia. You would expect to find a **right superior** quadrantanopia due to the proximity of the inferior optic radiation to Wernicke area in the left temporal lobe. Wernicke's is due to a lesion in the posterior temporal gyrus of the dominant hemisphere.

Board Testing Point: Recognize the clinical features of Wernicke aphasia.

578. Answer: D

Answer: ESR.
Use of screening tests in dementia workups are generally controversial—except when the tests are simple and inexpensive, and the etiology is a potentially reversible cause of dementia. The 4 other tests listed are easy to do and relatively inexpensive. They are helpful in ruling out infectious (RPR), metabolic (lytes, vitamin B_{12}), and endocrine (TSH) etiologies for dementia. The ESR is not a specific test helpful for defining a cause of dementia.

Board Testing Point: Know common laboratory tests to consider in the workup of dementia.

579. Answer: C

Answer: Obsessive-compulsive disorder.
This disorder frequently begins in adolescence or early adulthood. Note the excessive handwashing and "door checking"—this is classic for this disorder. Treatment with selective serotonin reuptake inhibitors (SSRIs) or clomipramine may be effective.

Board Testing Point: Recognize the clinical features of obsessive-compulsive disorder.

580. Answer: C

Answer: Sodium bicarbonate.
Sodium bicarbonate helps by alleviating depression of the sodium-dependent channel. Naloxone is a treatment for narcotic overdose. Physostigmine and phenytoin are not effective. Flumazenil is contraindicated because it will reduce the seizure threshold.

Board Testing Point: Recognize the clinical utility of using sodium bicarbonate in a tricyclic antidepressant overdose.

581. Answer: E

Answer: N-acetylcysteine + activated charcoal.
This patient has an acetaminophen overdose. Hepatotoxicity is less when N-acetylcysteine is combined with activated charcoal (25% hepatotoxicity with N-acetylcysteine alone vs. 4% when it is combined with activated charcoal).

Board Testing Point: Know the antidote and therapy for acetaminophen overdose.

582. Answer: A

Answer: No further testing; begin antibiotics.
This elderly patient is admitted for surgical treatment of hip fracture and develops delirium and fever postoperatively. She has a nonfocal exam and most importantly an abnormal U/A, suggesting UTI as the cause of delirium. Nosocomial meningitis is extremely rare, especially if the patient has not had a neurosurgical procedure. If the patient has evidence of infection (pneumonia, UTI, skin), then treatment of the infection is the appropriate course. Workup of a CNS infection is not necessary unless no alternative site of infection is found. Delirium and mental status changes are very common in the elderly when they develop infections.

Board Testing Point: Recognize UTI as a common cause of delirium in the elderly.

583. Answer: B

Answer: *Acanthamoeba*.
Acanthamoeba can cause amebic keratitis. It occurs in normal hosts and causes a chronic inflammation of the cornea. Almost all cases occur in contact lens wearers. Patients will present with "foreign-body" sensation and severe pain. Blurred vision and photophobia are common. Annular infiltration also occurs. Diagnosis is by finding the trophozoite form or cysts in corneal scrapings or biopsy. The key for this question was that he was a contact lens wearer who had poor lens hygiene. *Staphylococcus epidermidis*—think about this after ocular surgery, particularly cataract extraction or lens implantation. *B. cereus* occurs after penetrating eye trauma, and is one of the few organisms that will give you a ring abscess; *Pseudomonas* and *Proteus* are about the only other 2 bacteria that will do that as well. *Bartonella henselae*—no kitties around in the history, and usually you'll get a conjunctivitis picture, **not** this nasty scenario.

Board Testing Point: Know that *Acanthamoeba* is a likely organism found in a contact lens wearer with a severe eye infection.

584. Answer: D

Answer: Carotid duplex.
This patient has the sudden onset of right eye visual loss. He has a history of diabetes but no history of retinopathy or evidence of retinopathy on the funduscopic exam. The diabetes is a major risk for vascular disease; the funduscopic finding of a "cherry red spot" is consistent with retinal artery occlusion. The most likely cause of this would be atherosclerotic plaque emboli from a diseased carotid artery. The most appropriate first diagnostic test would be a carotid duplex. If surgery is possible based on results of a carotid duplex, a carotid angiogram would be a reasonable secondary test prior to an endarterectomy. Head CT scan or MRI would not be diagnostically helpful in this case.

Board Testing Point: Recognize the clinical features of retinal artery occlusion and the need to evaluate with a carotid duplex.

585. Answer: B

Answer: Pituitary tumor.
Chiasmal lesions interrupt the central fibers that mediate temporal vision—therefore, a pituitary tumor, or craniopharyngioma, results in loss of visual fields in the bitemporal regions. If the lesion was posterior to the chiasm—such as loss of visual cortex in 1 occipital lobe—a complete loss of visual perception in one field would result.

Board Testing Point: Recognize the clinical features of a chiasmal lesion.

586. Answer: E

Answer: Left sympathetic chain.
The symptoms are consistent with sympathetic denervation of her left eye—the "Horner" pupil. Most commonly, pulmonary neoplasms of the superior sulcus will produce this lesion. Usually "Horner" pupil is associated with ipsilateral ptosis and anhidrosis. Pupillary light responses should be normal, as should the response to agents that dilate and constrict the pupil. However, since the sympathetic chain is not working, cocaine cannot cause local release of sympathomimetic substances and is a poor dilator.

Board Testing Point: Recognize the clinical features of "Horner" pupil and that there must be a problem in the ipsilateral sympathetic nerve.

587. Answer: D

Answer: Presbyopia.
This is the normal aspect of aging that occurs between the ages of 40 and 50. The lens slowly loses its ability to accommodate for near vision. Patients usually need bifocals or reading glasses for near vision.

Board Testing Point: Recognize the clinical manifestations of presbyopia.

588. Answer: D

Answer: Glaucoma.
This patient has noticed some visual changes. On funduscopic exam, she has a high cup-to-disc ratio suggestive of glaucoma. A normal cup-to-disc ratio is usually less than 1:2. The retinal exam does not show hemorrhages or exudates that would be expected in a patient with advanced hypertensive retinopathy. This patient is much younger (58) than is usually seen with macular degeneration.

Board Testing Point: Recognize the clinical features of glaucoma.

589. Answer: C

Answer: Cytomegalovirus retinitis.
This patient has advanced HIV disease with a very low CD4 count (26). Almost all individuals who develop CMV retinitis have CD4 counts less than 50. He has typical symptoms of CMV retinitis (floaters). His funduscopic exam shows large hemorrhages and exudates consistent with CMV retinitis. HIV retinopathy is asymptomatic, and on funduscopic exam, cotton wool spots are seen. Retinal TB is much less common than CMV, and would be even less likely with the patient on active antituberculous therapy. *Cryptococcus* rarely ever involves the retina. Toxoplasmosis is a possibility but is far less common than CMV retinitis.

Board Testing Point: Recognize in a patient with HIV and low CD4 count that CMV retinitis is the most likely etiology of visual disturbances.

590. Answer: B

Answer: Subcutaneous low-molecular-weight heparin injections.
Warfarin is absolutely contraindicated in pregnancy, so those answer options should be thrown out. Thrombolytics would also be reserved for very hemodynamically unstable patients. Heparin is also **not** without risks, but the risks are much greater that she will have recurrent pulmonary embolisms without it.

Board Testing Point: Recognize that warfarin is contraindicated during pregnancy.

591. Answer: D

Answer: Urine culture, HIV ELISA, and RPR.
Most states require RPR testing, and many are recommending that HIV ELISA testing also be done. Urine culture is always done initially, because asymptomatic bacteruria is quite common in pregnancy, and these women have an increased risk of pyelonephritis and other infections. HSV II serology is essentially worthless. The main factor in determining if a woman is at risk for transmission of HSV is the presence of active lesions at the time of delivery—if present, then she would undergo a C-section. Other tests done at the initial visit usually include: Rh-type, hematocrit/hemoglobin and MCV, cervical cytology, rubella immunity testing, hepatitis B testing, *Chlamydia* screening, and thyroid function.

Board Testing Point: Know what tests to order for screening in a pregnant woman.

592. Answer: C

Answer: Begin a trial of an oral contraceptive agent.
Irregular bleeding with intervals less than 18 days indicates a luteal phase abnormality. This can usually be alleviated with the use of oral contraceptives. If she had prolonged bleeding with normal intervals, then you would be concerned about submucosal fibroids. Other factors to consider in excessive or abnormal bleeding are spontaneous abortion or ectopic pregnancy. Medical causes of dysfunctional bleeding include hypothyroidism, liver disease with resultant coagulopathy, thrombocytopenia, and chronic renal failure.

Board Testing Point: Recognize the clinical utility of a trial of oral contraceptives in a woman with irregular menstrual bleeding.

593. Answer: C

Answer: Endocervical polyp.
Of those things listed, polyp is the most likely anatomic abnormality. Frequently, though, the examination will be normal.

Board Testing Point: Recognize the clinical features associated with an endocervical polyp.

594. Answer: E

Answer: Endometriosis.
Patients usually are nulliparous and over 30 with the following symptoms: dysmenorrhea, dyspareunia, dyschezia, and/or perimenstrual spotting. The most common site is the ovaries (look for tender adnexa in an afebrile patient).

Board Testing Point: Recognize that endometriosis is a common cause of infertility.

595. Answer: A

Answer: Pregnancy test.
Don't forget that pregnancy is a common presentation for primary amenorrhea in teenagers! Teen pregnancy is a rampant problem in the U.S., and primary amenorrhea will commonly present this way!

Board Testing Point: Remember that pregnancy is a common reason for amenorrhea in adolescents.

596. Answer: B

Answer: Semen analysis.
Here the answer is to go for cheap, easy, and relatively noninvasive. Infertility is a "male" problem 1/3 of the time. Normal semen has the following properties: ejaculate volume > 1 mL; sperm concentration > 20 million/mL; initial forward motility > 50% of sperm; normal morphology > 60% of sperm.

Board Testing Point: Recognize that in over 1/3 of cases of infertility, male infertility issues are the cause.

597. Answer: D

Answer: Continue with current regimen.
This woman has HIV and had a low CD4 count and high viral load before starting on highly active antiretroviral therapy. The correct approach is to continue treating the patient with a very active regimen. This will maintain the best immune system for this patient and keep the chance of transmission to the baby minimal (likely 1% or less). Zidovudine alone has been studied and lowers transmission rate to 8%, compared to about 30% without zidovudine. However, single-drug therapy with zidovudine would not be appropriate because resistance would likely develop—and it would not protect the woman's immune system as well as her current regimen. Zidovudine alone is also not as effective as a 3-drug regimen in reducing transmission. There is no reason to switch to a different, potentially more toxic regimen (ddI/d4T/amprenavir). Cases of lactic acidosis occurring during pregnancy have been reported in women on d4T. The combination of d4T and ddI increases the risk of neuropathy in the patient. Efavirenz is contraindicated during pregnancy. Nevirapine is also avoided if her CD4 count is > 250 because of poor outcomes.

Board Testing Point: Know that for pregnant women with HIV, you should use antiretroviral therapy to reduce viral load to undetectable levels.

598. Answer: C

Answer: Continue on the OCP, intensify insulin regimen for target glycated Hb 6.
This woman with Type 1 DM wishes to become pregnant. She should have tight control of her diabetes during pregnancy, and it's especially important during the 1st trimester. She should work intensively at lowering her glycated Hb **before** getting pregnant. Target glycated Hb is 6.0. The risks of tight control in the pregnant woman include increased risk of hypoglycemia, and ironically, tighter control in pregnancy increases risk of worsening diabetic retinopathy.

Board Testing Point: Recognize the clinical utility of strict glucose control before becoming pregnant.

599. Answer: B

Answer: Kegel exercises.
This patient has symptoms typical of stress incontinence (episodes occurring when she laughs, sneezes, or coughs). Medications rarely work for this kind of incontinence. Kegel exercises are exercises by which patients strengthen the pelvic floor muscles, which can help with urethral control of urine flow. Some patients with stress incontinence may need surgery to reposition the bladder.

Board Testing Point: Recognize that Kegel exercises are the treatment of choice for stress incontinence and that pharmaceutical therapy is generally ineffective.

600. Answer: B

Answer: 69-year-old healthy woman with essential hypertension taking HCTZ.
The U.S. Public Health Service task force recommends DXA scanning for women beginning at age 65 unless there is 1 risk factor in addition to menopause. A man should have the first DXA scan at age 70 in the absence of risk factors. Prominent risk factors which necessitate an earlier DXA scan include glucocorticoid use, history of eating disorder, hyperparathyroidism, malabsorption, thyrotoxicosis, and anticonvulsant use. A DXA scan done in a young woman is not predictive of osteoporosis. The humeral fracture was related to high impact trauma and is not a fragility fracture. In individuals with normal thyroid function, there is no increased risk of bone loss.

Board Testing Point: Know when to order a DXA scan.